Juicing For Beginners

Best Juice Cleanse Diets for Weight
Loss and Detox in Just 7 Days. Learn
About the Benefits of Fasting, Juicing,
and Ways to Improve Your Health,
Mind, and Body

David Green

Table of Contents

Introduction: Juice, Anyone?

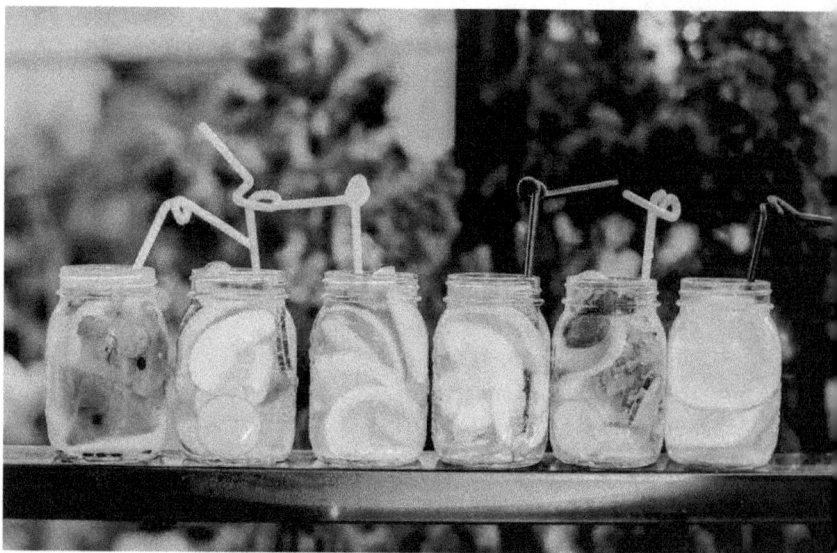

Fig. 1: Juice. Unsplash, by Kaizen Nguyễn, 2017, https://unsplash.com/photos/jcLcWL8D7AQ/
Copyright 2017 by Kaizen Nguyễn/Unsplash.

"Breakfast without orange juice is like a day without sunshine." (Bryant)

How often do you drink juice?

I don't mean the boxed, bottled or processed varieties, but glasses of juice made from fresh, whole, and healthy ingredients. If you love drinking juice, then this eBook will surely prove useful to you as it is all about how you can get the most out of this refreshing drink. If you don't drink juice or you don't make your own juice at home, now is the time to start.

These days, food has become so varied and abundant that a lot of people end up overindulging frequently. Processed meat products, high-sugar pastries, junk foods, fast foods, and more. As you keep eating these kinds of foods, you may notice yourself gaining weight and developing a number of troubling health issues. Because of this, you would look for ways to detoxify and 'reset' your body to improve your health.

If you are reading this eBook, it means that you have realized that it's time for you to start changing your habits. This is a great thing! Now, the next step is to determine how you can start on the path towards a healthier body.

For this, juicing might just be the key to unlock a healthier you.

While juicing may seem simple and easy, there's more to it than most people think. For one, juicing comes with a bunch of health benefits that you will surely be interested in. Here are some examples:

- Juicing helps you increase your fruit and veggie intake per day.
- Juicing allows you to consume a lot of nutrients that your body will absorb easily.
- Juicing offers detoxifying effects to make you healthier.
- Juicing promotes weight loss.
- Juicing gives you more energy.
- Juicing is simple, easy, and it offers a lot of variety.
- Juicing is suitable for adults and children too—although the juicing methods may vary according to age.
- Juicing gives your immune system a boost.
- ... and so much more!

This is just a sneak peek of the wonderful things you can look forward to when you start juicing. Later, we will discuss these benefits in detail. Of course, this isn't the only thing you will learn about juicing in this eBook. Here, you will discover everything there is to know about juicing such as what juicing is all about, the things to keep in mind if you are planning to start, finding the best juicer for your needs, preparing the equipment and ingredients to start juicing, how to juice for weight loss, the perfect types of juice for the different aspects of your health, and so much more. You will even learn a number of recipes in this eBook that are simple, tasty, and healthy.

By the end of this eBook, you will have a better understanding of what juicing is truly about and how you can start your own juicing plan safely. One of the best things about juicing is that it's completely customizable. Although you will learn a bunch of tips and guidelines here, at the end of the day, you would have to come up with your own plan of action. Figuring out what is best for you will allow you to enjoy all the benefits of juicing while making it sustainable—and you will learn everything you need to do this right here.

But before we continue, I would like to tell you my story and why I have decided to write this eBook. All my life, I have been dealing with weight issues. I am now in my 40s but while I was growing up, I had dealt with problems like hypertension, metabolic issues, and constant swings between weight loss (which made me feel happy) and weight gain (which often made me feel like a failure). When I reached the ripe age of thirty, I told myself that it was time to make a change. I didn't want to have to deal with weight issues for the rest of my life so I started researching.

As I was researching, I discovered juicing and I was hooked ever since. For more than a decade, I have learned everything I can about juicing. I had also worked hard to perfect the best juicing recipes to help shed excess pounds and maintain a healthy weight long-term. Apart from this, I also learned the best types of juices and juice recipes that helped me overcome some of my chronic health problems. Juicing has allowed me to focus more on my nutrition and through this, I discovered the most effective holistic solutions that actually work.

After doing research, I applied everything I learned. I evolved from a juicing beginner to a juicing master. Over the past few years, I had also studied new juicing ingredients, recipes, and equipment to refine the process and get the most out of it. After years of studying this concept, applying my knowledge, and coming up with my own tips and strategies, I felt experienced enough to share what I know with others... and so I wrote this eBook.

Teaching other people all about juicing is important to me because it is the one thing that I attribute my health improvements to. I have tried so many methods in the past and yet, none of them seemed to work for me. But through juicing, I have become happier and healthier. Because of this, I believe that other people—yes, even you!—can get the same great results with the right knowledge and guidance. As someone who has tried, tested, and succeeded in juicing, I can promise you that everything you will learn in this eBook will help you become a juicing master too. As time goes by, you will start noticing the many benefits that juicing has to offer.

When it comes to making changes for your health, you must focus on the decisions that you make. Always remember that you will be making those decisions for yourself and for your health. You are not deciding for anyone else and you should never base your decisions on the impossible standards of society. While juicing is simple enough, you shouldn't go all-in right away. Making drastic restrictions is never the way to go!

Instead, you should ease into juicing gradually to make the journey easier for you. Choose recipes that you love so that you will be excited to enjoy your homemade juice time and time again. This is especially important at the beginning of your juicing journey. If you slip up once in a while, that's okay. As long as you keep your end goal in mind, you will always find ways to motivate yourself to keep going.

Juicing is healthy. Juicing is fun. Juicing will improve your health and your life in more ways than one. If you're ready to embark on a healthier lifestyle, turn the page, and let's begin...

Chapter 1:

All About Juicing

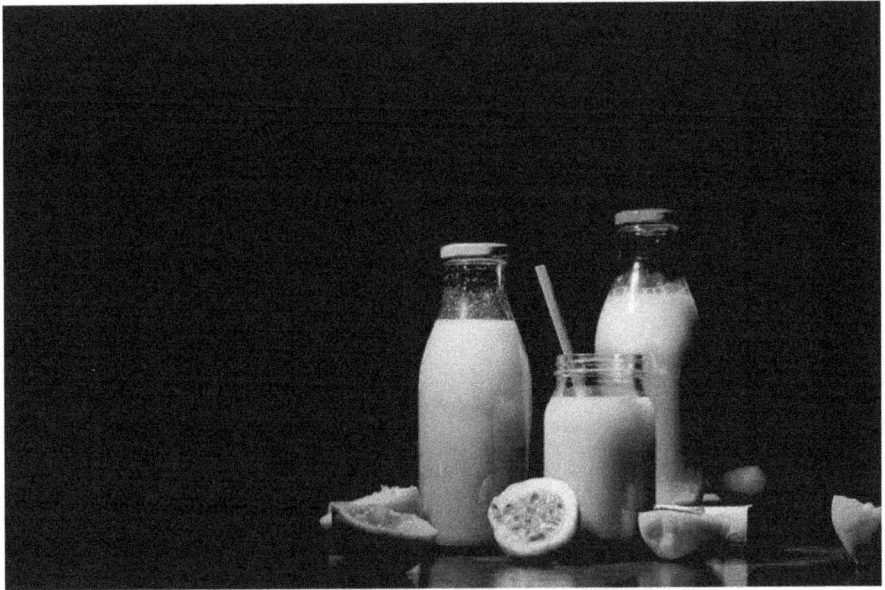

Try keying in the term 'juicing' on a search engine and you will surely find tons of results. When it comes to juicing, there is a ton of information available, however, this method remains to be somewhat misunderstood.

As someone interested in juicing, do you know what it is, what it entails, and what are the health benefits that it offers? If not, you don't have to worry because we will clarify everything here in the first chapter before we move on to the 'how' of juicing.

If you have ever tried researching health and fitness, you would have already established that fruits and veggies are good for your health. This, of course, is a fact. Fresh produce can help prevent the risk of developing diseases, can give you higher energy levels, and even improve your skin—and these are just some of the health benefits that fruits and veggies have to offer. This is one of the main reasons why people all over the world are becoming interested in plant-based diets.

So... what does this have to do with juicing?

Juicing is a process wherein you extract healthy and nutrient-dense juices from fresh vegetables and fruits. This should be very clear—juicing involves the extraction process. When you start juicing, it doesn't mean that you will buy processed fruit juices from supermarkets and drink these throughout the day. These products are typically laden with sugars and other unhealthy ingredients, which means that they aren't good for you. Instead, you will be making your own fresh juice at home using fruits, vegetables or tasty combinations of both fruits and veggies.

In recent years, juicing has grown in popularity as a way for people to increase their fruit and veggie intake or for the purpose of detoxifying their bodies. Whatever your reason is for wanting to go on a juice cleanse or a juicing journey, it's important to focus only on fresh ingredients when making your juices.

Since the process of juicing extracts the healthy liquid from fruits and veggies, it typically removes all solid matter such as pulp, seeds, and skin. By using a juicer, you will be able to extract liquid that contains almost all of the nutrients, vitamins, and minerals of the produce you juice. This means that you can drink all of that yummy, healthy goodness without having to eat whole fruits or veggies.

Juicing isn't just a diet fad. In fact, it isn't even a diet. Instead, it's a wonderful way for you to improve your health. Although you can juice fruits like oranges and lemons by hand, it would be better for you to invest in a high-quality juicer, especially if you plan to go on regular juice cleanses. Later, we will be discussing the different types of juicers along with a couple of great products that are available at the time of writing this eBook. Now that you know the true definition of juicing, we will be delving into the different aspects of this healthy, easy process. By the end of this eBook, you will be able to start juicing for your health and happiness.

Answering the Most Common Question

Juicing is a healthy process that allows you to incorporate more fruits and veggies into your diet. Drinking fresh juice is easy, convenient, and you have countless options to choose from. As you juice fresh fruits and veggies, you will also be extracting the nutrients that the whole fruits contain. The juice that you extract is rich in healthy goodness and when you drink it, that goodness goes into your body too.

Just like me, proponents of juicing believe that it is a lot healthier to drink juice extracted from fresh produce than it is to eat the fruits and veggies whole. This is because juice already comes in a liquid form which means that your body can absorb it easily. Instead of having to work hard to digest the solid fruits and veggies, you will be giving your digestive system a much-needed break.

If you're not a fan of eating fruits and veggies (especially veggies), then I highly recommend that you start juicing. With all the wonderful benefits this process has to offer, you can't afford to not give it a try. Plus, we are still at the beginning of our book, which means that you have a lot more to learn. Before moving on, let's answer the most common question asked by people who are interested in juicing:

Should you juice or eat fruits and veggies as they are?

The answer to this is both. If you can, you should focus on eating fresh fruits and vegetables regularly. If you're not used to this, start by eating the kinds that are most palatable to you. As you get used to eating these healthy plant-based food sources, then you can start experimenting with more adventurous types of fruits and vegetables, those which you never thought you would try out.

Eating fresh fruits and vegetables will give your body fiber, vitamins, minerals, and nutrients to keep you strong and healthy. Of course, juicing has its own extensive range of advantages too, especially if you're not fond of eating fresh produce. You can start getting used to the fresh options by juicing first. You can also opt to eat the fresh fruits and vegetables that you like then supplement your diet by juicing, where you would use the fruits and veggies you're not used to eating as ingredients for your juice blends.

But it would also be beneficial for you to go on juice cleanses regularly to help 'reset' your body and make you healthier. Later, we will discuss juice cleanses in more detail. One thing you should know first is that there is a safe way to do a juice cleanse and you should know this to ensure that you don't compromise your health in any way.

The Wonderful Benefits of Juicing

When done correctly, juicing is a fun, safe, and convenient way to live a happier and healthier life. Juicing offers a number of potential health benefits that you may enjoy as you make this process a regular part of your life. Let's take a look at some of the most significant benefits now. Later, I will share other benefits with you but for now, let's start with these:

Juicing Preserves the Nutritional Profiles of Fruits and Vegetables

Although eating fresh fruits and vegetables is good for your health, juicing them is ideal too as the process preserves the nutritional profiles of the produce. Whenever you juice fruits, veggies or both, you get a glass of fresh juice that contains more concentrated nutrients that your body absorbs easily. The reason for this is that generally, most of the nutrients found in fruits and vegetables are found in the juice—not in the fibrous material or pulp that you have to eat. Naturally, this makes it beneficial for your health.

According to one study, a diet that is rich in vegetables and fruits is typically associated with a decreased risk of developing chronic disease (Esfahani, A., et. al., 2011). Since juicing involves the use of these healthy food items, you can potentially improve your health so much that you will also reduce your risk of developing health issues. Juicing involves extracting juice from fresh produce, which means that you only get the "good stuff" sans the many sugars, preservatives, and additives that are typically mixed in with processed juice drinks.

Unless you are a vegetarian or your diet mainly consists of plant-based sources, chances are, you aren't able to consume the recommended daily amount of vegetables and fruits. But if you supplement your diet with fresh juices, then this will surely allow you to get all of the nutrients you need. Since you will be drinking the juice, you won't feel like you are forcing yourself to eat more than you want to. In fact, in a matter of weeks, you can already improve your body's nutrient levels if you can consistently make this process a part of your life. You will get essential nutrients like folic, vitamin E, selenium, vitamin C, beta carotene, and a huge boost in your body's antioxidant levels.

Apart from maintaining the nutritional profiles of fruits and veggies, juicing can even help your body absorb these nutrients more effectively. Whenever you consume something, your digestive system gets to work. But when it realizes that you have only consumed juice with no solids to break down, your body will be able to process this faster. This means that your body will also absorb the nutrient content of the juices faster and more effectively for the nutrients to go into the various systems in your body. Think about it: when nutrients start circulating in the different systems of your body in a matter of thirty minutes, isn't this much better than having to wait a couple of hours for your body to digest whole foods before distributing the nutrients to its different parts?

Of course, it is.

Through juicing, your body can absorb all of the nutrients from all of the ingredients you use for your fresh juices and juice blends. In other words, when you drink fresh fruit or vegetable juice, it is already 'pre-digested,' so your body can start using it right away. And the more fruits and vegetables you use, the more nutrients your body will enjoy.

Juicing is Gentler on Your Digestive System

This is one of the most significant benefits of juicing, especially if you're having problems with the consumption of too much fiber. As an advocate of juicing, I have personally experienced this benefit. Since juicing removes the hard-to-digest fiber from fruits and veggies, your digestive system doesn't have to work hard after you drink a refreshing glass of juice. In this form, your body absorbs all the "good stuff" more effectively too. For instance, your body gets higher levels of the beneficial carotenoid known as beta-carotene when you get it from juice rather than whole fruits and veggies.

If you suffer from certain malabsorptive conditions or diseases, you will benefit a lot from juicing as it fits into low-residue and low-fiber diets. Although research about this fact is still limited, there are plenty of anecdotal reports from people like me who attest to the benefit of healthier digestion through juicing.

When you drink a glass of juice, your body doesn't have to break down any solids, especially if you strain the juice first before drinking. This means that your digestive system doesn't have to initiate the chemical process it needs to break solid food down into a liquid. By juicing regularly, your digestive system will thank you for it as it doesn't have to keep working hard all day and all night to process all of the solid foods you eat each day, especially high-fiber foods like fruits and vegetables. If you're looking for something that is gentler on your digestive system, a glass of juice is a perfect choice.

In line with this benefit, juicing also allows you to balance your gut microflora. By drinking fresh juice, you can increase the health-promoting bacteria in your intestines. This is an important benefit since one study has shown that the health of your gut microflora can contribute to your overall health too (Henning, S., et. al., 2017). Juices made from fresh fruits and veggies contain fiber, nitrate, polyphenols, and oligosaccharides, all of which may induce a similar effect as probiotics. This another popular reason why more people are turning to juice cleanses to improve their health.

Juicing is an Excellent Way For You to Add More Fruits and Vegetables to Your Diet

If you're not very fond of fruits and vegetables, you can increase your intake through juicing. For a lot of people, this is the more 'appealing' way to consume fresh produce because they don't really like the taste, especially when it comes to vegetables. Then there is the very high recommended daily amount of fruits and veggies you should eat. If you try to reach this target, you will feel too full to eat anything else! Unfortunately, this isn't ideal because it might make you feel like you're restricting yourself from eating the foods you like. But when you drink a glass of healthy, fresh, and tasty juice, you won't even feel like you have consumed adequate amounts of essential nutrients. Even if you feel full after drinking a glass of juice (because of the high-fiber content), you would have enjoyed the beverage so you won't feel as bad.

Although the process of juicing eliminates some of the fiber from fresh fruits and vegetables, you can easily add it back in by adding some of the pulp left in your juicer. This will give your juice a bit of texture. If you don't mind drinking juice with some pulp in it, the juice you drink becomes even healthier. As you already know by now, you have the option to perform juice cleanses regularly to get all of the benefits of juicing or you can drink a few glasses of fresh juice each day to increase your fruit and veggie intake. This makes juicing a supplement to your diet that won't cause adverse side effects.

According to one study, many Americans aren't able to reach the recommended intake levels of micronutrients by simply eating their 'normal' meals (Fulgoni, V., et. al., 2011). But when you add juicing to your daily regimen, you can consume the nutrients you need without feeling too pressured. Since juices are made from natural ingredients, they are typically healthier and safer to consume than taking vitamin or mineral supplements to reach your recommended daily nutrient intake. Through juicing, you will be consuming more fruits and vegetables—especially if these foods aren't normally part of your diet.

When you think about it, juicing also improves your eating habits. As you get used to drinking fresh juice, you will eventually learn how to love the taste. And when you experience the different benefits of juicing, this will encourage you to keep going. Take my case, for instance. Because of juicing, I learned how to opt for healthy foods when I started to see myself shedding excess pounds. Now, the healthy diet I am following is just a normal thing for me. Even though I indulge in 'unhealthy' foods once in a while, I still go back to juicing. Simply knowing that I am getting enough fruits and veggies each day already makes me feel happy—and my body can feel the good effects too!

Juicing Allows You to Create Flavor Combinations That are More Palatable Than the Individual Ingredients

Juicing doesn't mean that you have to only extract fresh juice from a single fruit or vegetable. If I only had to drink plain cabbage or broccoli juice to get more vegetables in my diet, I might not have lasted long enough to lose weight and enjoy the other benefits. Another amazing benefit of juicing is that it offers endless possibilities and personally, this is one of my favorite benefits of juicing.

While it's easy to make juice from a single fruit or vegetable, you can go beyond this if you want to make things more interesting. By combining different fruits and veggies plus a few herbs, spices, and natural sweeteners, you can create incredible flavor combinations that are a lot more palatable than the individual ingredients. As you experiment with different ingredient combinations, you will also be adding more variety to your diet. Soon, you will even be trying fruits and veggies that you swore you would never eat.

As you will discover in the next chapters, juicing allows you to make different recipes according to your personal preferences and health goals. As you are starting out, you can mix and match ingredients that you like. But if you are trying to reach specific health goals like losing weight or preventing disease, for example, then you can look for recipes that will help you reach these goals. Typically, these recipes consist of specific fruits or vegetables that provide the benefit you are looking for. Naturally, when you combine the fruits and veggies that offer the same benefits, you will get juice blends that will help you reach your goals faster.

The more you practice juicing, the more you will learn how to create balanced, palatable flavors (unless you are following recipes). When it comes to creating tasty and healthy juices, the key here is to understand that some flavors will complement each other while others won't. For instance, contrasting flavors typically blend well together like mellow, sweet juices combined with highly acidic ones. To become a juicing master, you have to learn these things. Fortunately, you will learn easily as long as you are willing to try new things.

Juicing Helps Cleanse and Detoxify the Body

Aside from weight loss, detoxification is one of the most popular benefits of juicing, especially for those who perform regular juice cleanses. Your body has natural detoxifiers—your kidneys and liver. Even without juicing or doing regular juice cleanses, these organs work hard to detoxify your body naturally. But when your liver and kidneys are forced to work hard all the time because your diet mainly consists of unhealthy food, then you might start developing problems with these important organs. To avoid this, juicing can help give your kidneys and liver a break by providing a detoxifying benefit.

If you give juice cleanses a try, you will feel the effects after a minimum of three days. This is why the shortest juice cleanses last for three days. Consuming nothing but juices and juice blends for three whole days will help cleanse your body of toxins while giving your digestive system a break too. We will be discussing this benefit again later along with how to do a proper juice cleanse for the purpose of detoxification. For now, let me share some studies with you that illustrate the importance of juicing in terms of detoxification along with other amazing benefits.

One study has shown that consuming beetroot juice while following a low nitrate diet can help decrease your blood pressure (Coles, L. & Clifton, P., 2012). When this happens, it also reduces your risk of developing cardiovascular disease. In another study, the researchers discovered that beetroot and green, leafy vegetables have positive vascular effects on the body mainly because of their dietary nitrate content (Lidder, S., & Webb, A.,

2013). This means that you should start drinking juice blends that contain these ingredients if you want to enjoy this benefit.

In another study, the researchers discovered that polyphenols, a type of dietary antioxidant, can help reduce the oxidative damage in the brain that may lead to the development of Alzheimer's Disease. Fortunately, these polyphenols can be found in different vegetables and including them in your juices can help you get this benefit too. In a similar study, the researchers also discovered that regular intake of fruits, and veggies can help reduce the risk of developing chronic disease, especially in the elderly (Gibson, A., et. al., 2012). It may even give the immune function a boost.

When you think about it, these benefits are actually brought about by the detoxification properties of juicing. Since toxins are a significant contributing factor to the development of diseases, detoxifying your body regularly through juicing will surely improve your overall health.

Other Benefits

The benefits above are the most significant benefits that you can look forward to as you start juicing. However, these aren't the only ones. Depending on how often you juice, the types of juice you drink, and your approach to juicing, you may also experience the following benefits:

- **Increased Energy Levels**

  Since fruits and vegetables are rich in healthy nutrients, extracting their juices and combining them to create juice blends gives you an energy boost like no other. By choosing the right type of juice or juice blend to drink at the start of the day, you will have energy that will last for the whole day.

- **Maintain Adequate Levels of Hydration**

  Fruits and vegetables contain high levels of water. When you extract the juices from fresh produce, you will be able to maintain good hydration all day, every day.

- **Immune System Boost**

  The phytonutrient content of fruits and veggies gives them the ability to protect themselves against insects and ultraviolet light. When you consume these fruits and veggies, you will also be consuming the phytonutrients they contain. These are the ones that give your immune system a boost to keep you protected from different diseases.

- **Stress Relief and Improved Quality of Sleep**

  For this benefit, there is a specific vegetable I would recommend that you include in your juice blends—spinach. This green, leafy vegetable contains the essential amino acid called tryptophan that can produce serotonin. This is a chemical that helps improve the quality of your sleep by promoting a healthier sleep cycle, and it helps relieve stress too.

- **Enhanced Brain Power**

  When it comes to boosting brain health, there are so many types of fruits and veggies that do this such as grapes, apples, and spinach, to name a few. Even the options that are high in antioxidants can provide this important benefit. In particular, grapes help improve the communication between your brain cells while apples contain quercetin that protects the cells of your brain from the damage caused by free radicals.

- **Enjoy Healthier Skin and Hair**

  Juice extracted from fresh vegetables and fruits can help eliminate buildup from your tissues and blood. This is important as it restores the natural elasticity and alkalinity of your skin. In particular, juicing fruits and veggies with high water content like cucumbers will keep your skin healthy and hydrated.

  If you have issues like thinning hair or you have noticed your hair becoming more brittle, juicing may help ease these issues. Drinking juices made from fruits and veggies that are rich in vitamin B can stimulate hair growth by providing oxygen to your cells to improve the health of your hair follicles. Choosing fruits and veggies that are rich in vitamin A help prevent dandruff by stimulating oil production in your scalp.

- **Helps with the Management of Diabetes**

  Most people who suffer from diabetes develop this condition because of poor lifestyle choices, especially in terms of diet. But when you make changes to your diet by adding more fruits and veggies in the form of juice and juice blends, you may notice that managing your condition is much easier. By including fresh juice in your diet or by performing regular juice cleanses, you can improve your health enough to prevent diabetes from getting worse.

- **Make Your Eyesight Better**

  Vitamin A is important for the health of your eyes. If you are deficient in this vitamin, you might experience eye issues or worse, blindness. Drinking juices that are high in vitamin A can help you prevent eye infections and dry eyes. This vitamin can even prevent pink eye.

As you can see, juicing offers a variety of health benefits to make your life better. But the benefits don't stop here. In the next chapters, we will be discussing the other benefits in detail along with some of the best types of juice and juice blends that promote said benefits. But the bottom line is that juicing is convenient and amazingly good for your health.

A Few Key Things to Keep in Mind

With all of the benefits juicing has to offer, you might already feel excited to give it a try. But there are more benefits to look forward to, which we will discuss later. But if you want to perform juicing safely and successfully, there are some things you must keep in mind. Although juicing has the potential to initiate wonderful changes in your body, it's very easy to make mistakes that may end up causing adverse side effects to your body. To avoid these mistakes and ensure juicing success, here are a few things to be mindful of:

Watch Out For Sugar

To make juice blends more palatable, the easiest thing to do is add one type of fruit or two to the mix. If you can find fruits that help add to the nutritional value of the juice blends, even better! For instance, if you're making a green juice blend that promotes weight loss, you can add an apple or a few berries to make it sweeter. However, when it comes to adding fruits to your juice blends, you have to watch out for the total sugar content.

Try not to go overboard when adding fruits to your juices. Check the ingredients of the juice blends to see how much sugar they contain. When you constantly drink juices with high amounts of sugar you won't be able to achieve or maintain consistent energy levels. It's never a good idea to consume high amounts of sugar so this is one thing to be mindful of on your juicing journey.

Your Juicing Method Matters

The juicing method that you use or the way in which you extract juice from fresh fruit and vegetable matter, especially if you want to preserve the nutrient content of the ingredients you use. The juicing method you use depends on the juicer that you own. If you don't own a juicer yet but you are planning to buy one, you should learn about the different types to make sure that you get the right type of juicer for your needs.

Apart from the juicing method, another way to ensure juicing safety and success is to drink your juice the right away. Most of the time, freshly-made juices should be consumed right away since they aren't pasteurized. This means that these juices are more prone to bacterial growth, which may cause food poisoning. However, there are certain types of juices and juice blends that can be stored in the refrigerator. If you are following a recipe, check the notes to see if you can make a big batch and store the rest for a few days. If the recipe doesn't have such a note or if it specifically states that you should consume the juice right away, then this is what you should do.

Not All Juices are Created Equal

Just like all other beverages out there, not all juices are created equal. As you will discover when you start your juicing regimen, some juices are healthier than others. Some juices are tastier than others, some juices are more beneficial in terms of weight loss than others, and some juices provide more health benefits than others. This is why you should already know your health goals before juicing. Your personal health goals will help you determine what types of juice or juice blends you will make for yourself.

Also, freshly made juice is a lot healthier than processed juice. Although processed juices are much more convenient than juices that you make in your home, the extra effort you put into extracting juice from fruits and vegetables will be well worth it.

And if you can find the best recipes with the right ingredients, you will surely get the outcomes you desire in terms of health.

You Shouldn't Replace a Healthy, Balanced Diet with Juicing

Another very important thing to be mindful of when you start juicing is that you shouldn't use juicing as a replacement for a healthy, balanced diet. As mentioned, juicing can help supplement your healthy diet to increase your intake of fruits and veggies. You can also perform regular juice cleanses to detoxify and 'reset' your body for the purpose of improving your health.

But if you're interested in a 'diet' that will help you lose weight, juicing isn't the answer. If you only drink juice all day, every day, you will surely lose weight. If you are doing a juice cleanse, doing this for a few days up to a week will still be beneficial to your health. However, if you only consume juice and nothing else for months instead of following a healthy diet, you will surely experience adverse effects. Yes, you will lose weight, but not in a healthy or sustainable way. And once you start eating solid food, you will most likely regain all of the weight back—plus a few excess pounds.

When you try to use juicing as a fad diet to make you lose weight, this will potentially cause more harm than good. Unfortunately, a lot of people do this and when they start feeling the side effects, they think that juicing is to blame or juicing doesn't work. But the problem isn't with juicing. Rather, it's how people use juicing in an extreme way. In line with this, another risk you should know when it comes to juicing as a 'diet' is that it can even slow your metabolism down since you won't be eating any fat, protein or any other solid food. When this happens, your metabolism slows down and the bad part is, when you go back to your normal diet, you will be doing so with a slower metabolism. Naturally, this will cause you to gain weight.

The bottom line is that juice isn't an adequate replacement for meals unless you are doing a juice fast or a juice cleanse. Even if you plan to do a juice fast, you will also have to prepare for it to ensure that you do it properly and safely. Apart from this, juicing is meant to supplement your diet, enhance your meals to reduce your food intake (especially unhealthy foods), and you can also drink juice as a snack instead of munching on a bag of chips. These are the best ways to make the most out of juicing for the improvement of your health.

You Should Know the Risks

While juicing is very beneficial, it also comes with its own set of risks apart from the ones shared in the last point. Before I started juicing, I learned all about it, especially the risks. By being aware of the possible risks, you can protect yourself from them. Also, knowing these risks enables you to identify them in case you start experiencing them while juicing, especially when you're on a juice cleanse. In such a case, you should transition back into your normal diet then give your body time to adjust. After a week or two, you can give juice cleansing a try again.

Don't worry, we will discuss this more later. For now, here are the most common risks associated with juicing that you must be aware of:

- **Swings in blood sugar levels**

    Since most juice blends contain fruits, adding too many of these sweet foods can cause major swings in your blood sugar levels. This makes it very risky and even harmful to those who suffer from diabetes. This is why you should watch the sugar content of your juices and juice blends. As much as possible, try to stick with the juice blend recipes. If you really don't like the taste of a certain juice blend, give yourself time to adjust. As time goes by, juicing becomes easier and you'll stop craving for beverages that contain too much sugar.

- **Dysfunction of the GI tract**

Since most of the fiber of fruits and vegetables is extracted in the juicing process, this might be problematic for you, especially if you use juices to supplement your diet. If you don't eat any fruits and vegetables at all and you only rely on juices to get fiber in your diet, you might start experiencing GI tract dysfunction.

If you are doing a juice cleanse, you don't have to worry about this risk because your digestive system won't have to work hard to break down solid foods. However, if you eat a lot of unhealthy food and you only consume fruits and veggies in the form of juice, this will slow your digestion process down. This can have long-term effects since your GI tract is like your muscles—if it isn't being used well, it will start losing its function. In some cases, it might even shut down! Avoid this by learning how to balance your diet and use juicing properly.

- **Not getting enough calories**

Now that you understand what juicing truly entails, you should know that it is very low in calories. This becomes a risk if you use juicing the wrong way as mentioned in the last point. If you don't get enough calories to keep your body going, your metabolic processes might shut down. Even if you try researching different diets, you will see that they don't recommend going low-calorie as this can cause a number of side effects.

- **Protein deficiency**

  Although many vegetables and some fruits contain protein, their protein content isn't enough to keep your body healthy. Without enough protein in your body, it won't be able to eliminate toxins. This is okay while you're on a juice cleanse. But again, if you are supplementing your diet with juicing, make sure you are following a healthy, balanced diet to complement the juices you are drinking.

- **Deprivation and restrictive eating**

  Personally, I love juicing whether I am on a juice cleanse, I drink juice as a snack or I drink juice before meals to help me feel satisfied even with a smaller meal portion. But if you use juicing in an extreme and unhealthy way, you will feel deprived. Pushing yourself to only drink juice means that you will be practicing restrictive eating—which is both harmful and unhealthy. If you do this, you will start seeing juicing as a negative thing and you might give up on it even before you can benefit from it.

- **Other potential risks**

  Aside from the risks mentioned above, juicing comes with other potential risks such as:

  - Juicing might not be suitable for those who suffer from kidney disorders. Some types of juice and juice blends might be high in an acid known as oxalate. This acid can contribute to the formation of kidney stones and the development of kidney problems.

- If the juice cleanse that you do includes a method of bowel stimulation, you might end up losing too many valuable nutrients. This may lead to an imbalance in your electrolyte levels and even dehydration. This is why it's important to learn how to do juice cleanses properly so that you can avoid this risk.
- If you aren't able to drink your juice right away, this might make you susceptible to food poisoning and other illnesses. This is especially true if you have a weakened immune system.

You may have noticed that all of these risks only have a high likelihood of occurring if you don't learn how to juice properly. Fortunately for you, this eBook will provide you with everything you need to stay safe while juicing. The final point to consider, which also happens to be the most important one is:

Consult with Your Doctor First

Whether you are at the peak of your health or not, you should speak with your doctor first before you start juicing, especially if you plan to give juice cleanses a try. This becomes even more important if you suffer from any kind of medical condition. Since juicing comes with potential risks, consulting with your doctor gives you a chance to raise your concerns and ask for tips from your doctor. While you will learn a wealth of information here, it is still safer to have a conversation with your doctor about your plans to start juicing. Remember—your health should be your number one priority. After all, you wanted to learn more about juicing so that you can improve your health, right?

Chapter 2:

Finding the Perfect Juicer

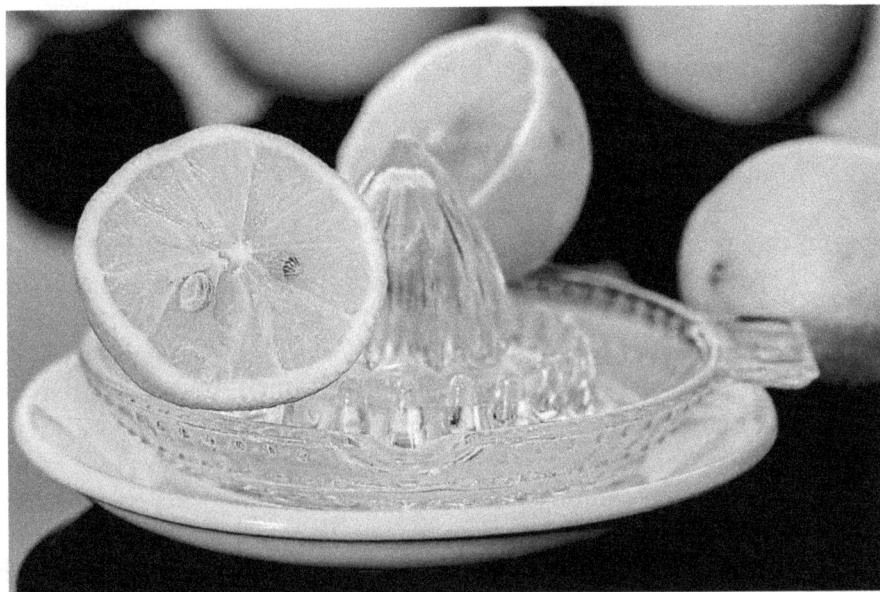

If you're planning to include juicing in your daily routine, the most important equipment that you must have is a high-quality juicer. If you want to extract juice from fresh fruits and vegetables regularly, finding the perfect juicer is key. After all, it can be very difficult and exhausting to try juicing fresh produce by hand each time. With a good juicer, the process of juicing becomes easier. Then all you have to do is gather your ingredients, prepare them, and start juicing!

Different Types of Juicers

If you already own a juicer, this chapter will be very useful for you as it will help you determine whether your juicer is the right one or not. If you don't own a juicer yet, this chapter will be even more useful as it will help you decide which is the best one to invest in. When it comes to juicers, there is no 'perfect' one. This is because the best juicer for you to choose would depend on your own needs and preferences. For instance, if you are a beginner and you only want to use juicing to supplement your diet, the juicer you choose will be very different from the model you would choose if you want to become a hardcore juicer who also does juice cleanses regularly.

Before investing in a juicer, you should know what you need. Although there are a few main types of juicers, these can be further broken down depending on the unique attributes and special features they possess. Also, juicers come in a wide range of prices. Naturally, the high-quality, powerful models that come with additional features are much more expensive than the simple juicers that don't come with bells and whistles. Juicers might seem like simple kitchen appliances but if you're serious about juicing, you should invest in one that will make you happy and help you reach your goals. To find the best one, the first thing you need to know is the different types of juicers you can choose from.

Centrifugal Juicers

Centrifugal juicers have tiny teeth and a basket that spins rapidly. These types of juicers will grind up fresh produce to give you fresh, pulpy juice. Then the juice will pass through a sieve with a fine mesh. Although centrifugal juicers work quickly and efficiently, you typically end up with a glass of juice with a lot of foam. If you're not into foamy beverages, a centrifugal juicer might not be your best choice. Also, you would have to drink the juice right away to avoid further oxygenation.

Sometimes, centrifugal juicers are classified as 'extractors' because of how they work. Also, since this type of juicer leaves a lot of pulp, you might end up wasting a lot of fresh produce if you simply throw the pulp away. If you're planning to go organic, a centrifugal juicer might be too wasteful for you. That is unless you will include the pulp in your juice or use it in some other way instead of throwing it out.

Centrifugal juicers are fast, but they are quite loud. If you live alone, this might not be an issue. However, if you have kids at home and you're planning to make fresh juice in the morning, the noise that this juicer makes might be a problem for you. This type of juicer is great for juicing hard fruits and veggies like apples and carrots although it might not be as effective for juicing leafy greens like kale and spinach. Centrifugal juicers are user-friendly, lightweight, and very easy to clean. After using the juicer, you can disassemble it and place the detachable parts in your dishwasher. Another benefit of centrifugal juicers is that they are typically the most affordable.

Citrus Juicers

As the name implies, citrus juicers are specifically meant for juicing oranges, lemons, and other citrus fruits. These types of juicers can either be electric or manual. Electric citrus juicers use a motor for spinning the reamer while manual citrus juicers have a handle for you to press the fruit against a grater. There are also commercial-grade citrus juicers that can either be electric, manual or fully automatic. Typically, these are more expensive but they also have high-quality parts.

Using a citrus juicer is very simple. All you have to do is cut the fruit horizontally, place it in the juicer, and extract the juice.

While a manual citrus juicer works well, electric and automatic citrus juicers are much easier to use.

Masticating Juicers

Masticating juicers get their name from how they work. These types of juicers mimic the 'chewing' of fruits and veggies as they have augers with sharp teeth made of metal. Unlike the centrifugal juicers, masticating juicers produce very little foam and they allow you to get the maximum amount of liquid from fresh produce, even from the pulp. Because the juicing process doesn't oxidize the liquid, you can make big batches of juice using this type of juicer then store the juice in your refrigerator. However, these juicers don't work as fast as centrifugal juicers.

Masticating juicers are also called "cold-press juicers" and you can use them to extract juice from kale, spinach, and other leafy greens. These types of juicers also work quietly and most people believe that they are more efficient at preserving the nutrient content of the ingredients juiced. Masticating juicers are more expensive than the other types and if you want one with a powerful motor, you have to pay for it. Another downside of this juicer is that you can't use it with citrus fruits and it's not very effective at juicing low-water veggies or fruits either.

Triturating Juicers

Triturating juicers have twin gears that rotate to crush fresh produce then grind it into fine particles. These powerful gears work efficiently to extract most of the juice from your ingredients until you are left with dry pulp and high-quality, nutrient-dense juice. Triturating juicers are especially effective at extracting juice from leafy greens, hearty veggies, and soft fruits. This type of juicer is relatively quiet but they are often bigger and bulkier than other types of juicers.

One huge benefit of these types of juicers is that you can use them for other tasks too, like chopping vegetables or grinding nuts and seeds. Since the juicer comes with added features, it also comes at a higher price. But if you plan to make different types of juices regularly and you want a piece of equipment that you can use for other purposes, this type of juicer may be the best option for you.

Horizontal or Vertical

Aside from these main types of juicers, you can also classify this piece of equipment as either vertical or horizontal. The choice you make would depend on the speed that you're looking for and the ingredients that you plan to juice. Horizontal juicers are ideal for juicing different types of fruits and veggies, even the dark and leafy kinds. These types of juicers are also quite versatile as you can use them to mince veggies or make pasta, nut butters, and sorbet. For some models, you would have to purchase extra attachments to do these additional tasks. Although highly efficient, horizontal juicers are quite slow. They are also more difficult to clean in general.

Of course, vertical juicers are the exact opposite of horizontal juicers. You can also use them to juice fruits and veggies, although not for juicing leafy, green veggies. Vertical juicers are smaller and faster too, making them a great choice if you plan to make juice every day or at every meal. However, they are generally noisier than horizontal juicers.

Juicer or Blender?

Although having a juicer will make your juicing process easier, you may opt for a high-quality blender too. You can make juice with blenders although the process may take longer because you have to strain the liquid first. Blenders will process all of the ingredients you put into them, which means that the final result will have a thicker texture. Blenders are ideal for making smoothies, soups, and pulpy juices. You can even add other ingredients to a blender such as seeds and nuts to create healthy, filling, and flavorful smoothies. If you do a juice cleanse, you can include smoothies in your schedule as long as you make sure that all of the ingredients have been processed finely. Blenders are very easy to clean too, especially when compared to some types of juicers.

If you already own a blender, you can supplement this by investing in a juicer. But if you don't own either of these kitchen appliances, then you have to think about which one to get for yourself. Since you're interested in juicing, then getting a high-quality juicer is recommended. To help you decide, you may want to think about the types of veggies or fruits that you want to include in your juicing journey. Also, think about whether you want to make smoothies or just juices and juice blends. At the end of the day, the decision lies with you.

But if you're interested in investing in a juicer, then there are some factors you need to consider to help you make the right choice. By choosing a juicer that suits your needs and preferences, your juicing journey will become easier and more sustainable. If you plan to get one of the more expensive models, make sure that it includes all of the features you need so that you don't end up wasting your hard-earned money on a piece of equipment you won't use. To help you decide, let's go through the most important factors for choosing the right juicer.

Step 1: What is Your Budget?

At this point, you already have an idea about the different types of juicers you can purchase. Now, it's time to make a decision. Choosing the right juicer is a process. Since you will be using the juicer to help improve your health, you want to make sure that the machine you choose will deliver. If you enjoy using the juicer, you will feel more motivated to stick with juicing and juice cleanses.

The first step you must take when choosing a juicer is to determine an optimal budget. Since there are different types of juicers to choose from, each with their own features, you can expect a wide range of prices too. For instance, you can get cheap juicers at $40 while some of the sturdier juicers with additional features can cost up to $1,600. Even if you plan to get a juicer somewhere between these two extreme price ranges, that would still be a significant amount of money so you should consider your juicer as an investment towards the improvement of your health.

To get the best juicer for your needs, you should first set a price range that you're comfortable with. This will make it easier for you to start searching for different juicers. For instance, if you go into a kitchen appliance shop and they offer you juicers that are well beyond your price range, you don't have to inspect them. Even better, you can directly ask the salespeople about juicers that fall within your budget. The same thing applies if you purchase your juicer online. When searching for a juicer in an online shop, you can set the filter to only show you juicers that fall within a specific price range.

Before setting your budget, think about your juicing needs. This will have an effect on the type of juicer you choose. For instance, if you mainly want to juice fruits, then you may opt for a centrifugal juicer which is generally cheaper. But if you are serious about juicing and you want to learn how to make complex and healthy recipes, then you have to look for a more versatile juicer. Even if you will spend more on it, you will be able to make all the juices and juice blends you need. And if you plan to do regular juice cleanses, such a juicer is more practical too.

The amount of money you are willing to invest in your juicer will depend on your own needs. You don't have to break the bank just to get a 'perfect' juicer because there is no such thing. Remember that the best juicer for you is one that will give you what you need, and one that will make you feel motivated to stick with your juicing journey, and, of course, one that you can afford. Take some time to think about your budget. Once you have decided on a price range for the juicer you will buy, you can move on to the next step in the process...

Step 2: Determine the Extraction Speed That You Need

The next step in your process of finding the best juicer is to research the speed of extraction you need. If you go back to the different types of juicers, this is one of the main features that make them different from one another. Generally, a slow extraction method is the better option because this speed won't generate heat. Unfortunately, heat tends to destroy some of the most beneficial ingredients in juices. This is something for you to ponder on. Although speed might seem like a good feature, it won't necessarily be beneficial for you.

The good news is that many juicers available on the market now offer multiple extraction speeds. This feature makes such juicers more versatile. Some juicers also offer different juicing modes for different kinds of ingredients—leafy vegetables, hard fruits, soft fruits, and so on. When choosing your juicer, make sure that it suits your needs. If you're always on-the-go and you plan to drink juice at every meal, then your best bet is a juicer that offers a high extraction speed. But if you don't mind a slower extraction speed, then you may opt for a juicer that works at a slower pace but gives you a more nutrient-dense glass of juice each time.

Of course, choosing a juicer that offers different extraction speeds would be the best but these come at a higher price. A juicer with multiple speed settings enables you to extract the highest amount of juice from different ingredients. With such a juicer, you can juice hard fruits and veggies at high speed and at low speed, you can juice soft fruits and veggies. This means that you can make different juice blend recipes to make your juicing journey more interesting. But if you have already set a budget and these types of juicers fall beyond the budget you have set, then you may have to settle for the next best thing. To do this, you can consider other factors too.

Step 3: Consider the Practical Factors

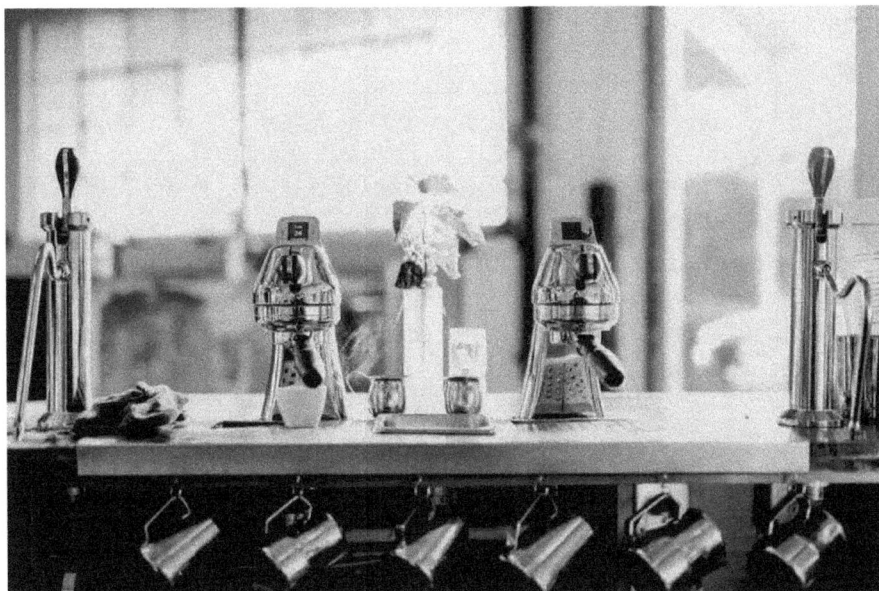

Fig. 4: Practical Features. Unsplash, by Nathan Dumlao, 2017,
https://unsplash.com/photos/vJiSzt85zZw/ Copyright 2017 by Nathan Dumlao/Unsplash.

The next step for you to take is to consider the more practical features of the juicer. When it comes to juicers and other kitchen equipment, practicality is very important. Even if you get a juicer at a very good price that offers the juicing speed you desire, if it's extremely complicated to use or it's very difficult to clean, you might give up on juicing after only a couple of weeks or months. When considering which juicers to buy, consider the following factors:

Cleaning

Cleanup is part of the juicing process, which means that it is something you would have to do after making your fresh juice or juice blend. To make the experience easier and more sustainable, you should choose a juicer that's easy to clean. Even if you haven't purchased a juicer yet, you can find this out already. There are many videos on YouTube where you can acquaint yourself with the construction of different juicer models. Through these videos, you can see what the different components look like and how many of these components you would have to wash after using the juicer.

Of course, it would take a lot of time for you to watch videos about every juicer on the market. Therefore, before you reach this step, you should already have a narrowed-down list of juicer models to choose from. Then all you have to do is learn more about the juicers on your list from how to clean them and all other practical factors.

Ease of Use

Aside from being easy to clean, the juicer you choose should also be easy to use, especially if you're a beginner. Opt for one that is easy to set-up, easy to take apart, and easy to clean. The ease of use will encourage you to keep using the juicer to improve your health. On the other hand, if you choose a model that's too complicated, just seeing it might cause you stress. When this happens, you might give up on your juicer and all the potential benefits you would have reaped through juicing.

Power

Just like the speed, the power your need for your juicer depends on the ingredients you plan to juice. For instance, if you want to juice a lot of hard fruits and veggies like apples and carrots, then you need a powerful juicer. The same thing applies if you want a heavy-duty juicer to use several times throughout the day. If you're serious about juicing and you want to make it a big part of your life, opt for a juicer with a powerful motor. That way, you won't have to change it after a few months of intense juicing.

Size

Another practical feature to consider is the size of the juicer. Make sure you have enough space in your kitchen countertop for the juicer you want to purchase. Ideally, you would place your juicer somewhere in your kitchen that's easy to access. There should be enough space to use the juicer and remove the parts easily when it's time to clean. If you have to move your juicer from one location to another every time you need to make juice, this might discourage you from using it regularly.

There are also some juicers that can be easily disassembled for storage. This would be a great option if you only plan to use the juicer for your regular juice cleanses. Then when you don't need it, you can simply store it somewhere in your kitchen until your next juice cleanse.

Spare Parts Availability

Finally, you should also consider the juicer's availability of spare parts. Although often overlooked, this is also an important factor so you won't have to replace your juicer if only one part malfunctions. After narrowing down your list of choices, check each of your options to see which ones have spare parts that are easy to find. This will help you narrow down your options even more.

Step 4: Remember That the Noise Level Matters, Too

Finally, check the noise level of the juicer too. This might not seem like a big deal right now, but if you happen to choose a juicer that works efficiently, fits into your budget, has all of the practical features you want, but makes too much noise, you might end up getting frustrated each time you use it. This is especially important if you live with your family. How can you enjoy a fresh glass of juice in the morning if making it will wake up your entire household?

The noise level of a juicer depends on how fast its motor is. Juicers with a high RPM of the motor will also produce high levels of noise while running. Think about your situation to help you determine whether you can deal with the noise or not. For instance, fast juicers like centrifugal juicers are very noisy but if you opt for a slower juicer like a masticating juicer, you won't have to deal with the noise. This is the final feature for you to consider when choosing your juicer. By the time you reach this feature, you should only have a few options left to choose from. And when you consider the noise level, you can already choose the best juicer for your needs.

Some of the Best Juicers on the Market Now

Lorem Now that you know how to choose the right juicer, it's time to share with you some of the best options available on the market on the writing of this book. Having to look at different juicers can be a time-consuming and exhausting task, especially if you have no idea where to start. To give you an idea of what great juicers look like, here are some of the most popular ones right now and the characteristics that make them great picks:

Breville JE98XL Fast Juicing Machine

This is a high-quality centrifugal juicer that offers an amazing combination of superior functionality and design at a reasonable price. The Breville JE98XL Fast Juicing Machine is one of the top sellers on Amazon because of all the amazing features it has to offer. This affordable juicer allows you to process fruits, veggies, and even roots effortlessly. It is a high-speed juicer that doesn't require a lot of preparation in terms of your ingredients. The best part is, the juice you make using this juicer stores well in the refrigerator for up to 48 hours without compromising its quality.

Effective and fast as this juicer is, it also comes with a few downsides. For one, it's not very efficient at juicing green, leafy veggies. It also makes quite a lot of noise while working because it has a very powerful motor that can juice ingredients in a matter of seconds. If these downsides are deal-breakers for you, that's okay. The Breville brand offers a wide range of incredible juicer models, some of which even offer multiple speed settings. If you're looking for a juicer to fit your needs, you can go through the different models this brand has to offer and start from there.

Hamilton Beach Easy Clean Big Mouth 2-Speed Juice Extractor

This juicer offers an optimal price to quality ratio, which makes it another great choice. With this juicer, you can get the most juice from various fruits and veggies like kale, oranges, and apples, for example. The Hamilton Beach Easy Clean Big Mouth 2-Speed Juice Extractor is an 800-watt appliance that comes with a 2-speed setting. It's an affordable juicer that's easy to use and easy to clean. If you're not yet willing to invest in an expensive model but you still want to have a versatile juicer, this is a great option.

Hurom HP Slow Juicer

As the name implies, this juicer works at a low speed. But it does come with heavy-duty strainers made of plastic and huge vertical grooves that are very easy to clean after juicing. The Hurom HP Slow Juicer features a tiled chamber for juicing that pours out more juice for you. With this juicer, you can make fresh-tasting juices and juice blends. With it, you can control how much pulp goes into your juice. It even comes with an ice cream and smoothie strainer, and a double-sided brush for cleaning.

Kuvings Whole Slow Juicer

This juicer features a feed tube with a wide mouth allowing you to juice different types of fruits and veggies with minimal preparation. It also comes with multiple strainers for smoothies, juice, and even ice cream. The Kuvings Whole Slow Juicer allows you to make smooth juice without pulp thanks to the extra-fine mesh strainer. It's easy to clean and it had a convenient carrying handle for easy portability.

Novis Vita Juicer

With this juicer, you can extract fresh juice from hard veggies and fruits. But it also comes with an additional attachment that allows you to ream citrus fruits too. The Novis Vita Juicer is a centrifugal juicer that works quietly at a low speed. With it, you can make pulpy juice or juice with no pulp depending on how you like your juice. This is a simple juicer with a large food tube, which means that you won't have to chop or dice your ingredients before juicing. It has a sleek design and it comes in an assortment of colors. However, if you plan to make big batches of juice, you may have to take a break once in a while to manually remove the pulp or fibrous leftovers to avoid clogging.

Omega J8006 Nutrition Center Masticating Juicer

This juicer has a powerful auger and motor so that you can cold-press huge amounts of juice from virtually any kind of produce. It is a compact juicer with sturdy construction and superior user-friendliness. The Omega J8006 Nutrition Center Masticating Juicer has parts that are dishwasher-safe making it very easy to clean. You can even use it as a food processor and a pasta maker. Talk about versatility! However, with this model, you have to chop or dice the ingredients first because of the small opening of its food chute. It is also one of the more expensive models available, but you won't be sorry because it offers superior performance in terms of juicing.

Oster JusSimple Easy Juicer Juice Extractor

This juicer has one of the best designs available. It's easy to clean and easy to use too. The Oster JusSimple Easy Juicer Juice Extractor features a rotating spout with close and open positions to ensure that the juice won't drip or leak from the food chute. It also features a wide mouth for minimal preparation before juicing. Because of all these features, this is a great option for beginners.

Tribest GSE-5050 Greenstar Cold Press

This juicer is affordable, efficient, and it's one of the most popular juicers available on the market. With this juicer, you can extract fresh juice from different ingredients while preserving the antioxidant and nutrient content of the fresh produce you use. The Tribest GSE-5050 Greenstar Cold Press features powerful twin gears along with a complete 3-stage juicing system. It even has a Reverse button that you can press in case you experience any tangling or clogging while you juice your ingredients. With this juicer, you can make fresh, nutritious juice with very little pulp. Although this is another expensive model, this is one of those juicers you can consider as a worthy investment. Even though it's quite bulky and it requires more maintenance, it's a solid machine that will serve you well if you plan to juice regularly.

As you can see, there are several models available for you to choose from. As long as you know what type of juicer you need and you follow the steps we discussed in this chapter, you will be able to find the best juicer for yourself. Then you can start using it to make fresh, healthy, and tasty juice.

Chapter 3:

Preparing What You Need

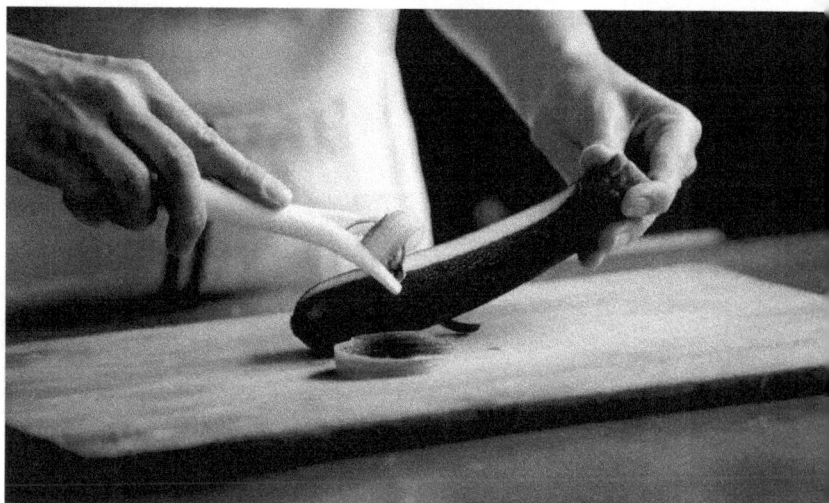

After finding the right juicer, it's time to learn how to prepare everything you need for each juicing session. Although pure juice made from a single type of fruit or vegetable is already healthy, you can make your juicing journey more interesting—and sustainable—by learning how to combine fruits and veggies. This is exactly what you will learn in this chapter. Here, you will discover the best types of fruits and veggies to use for juicing, as well as, the most challenging ones. You will also discover how to prepare your produce for juicing. Whether you already have a juicer or you have yet to choose one, this chapter will introduce you to the basics of juicing to help you succeed in this healthy endeavor.

The Best Juicing Options

Ideally, you should try to extract juice from all types of fruits and veggies. However, there are certain types of produce that are easy to juice and there are the ones that can be very challenging. The good news is that the easy ones outnumber the challenging ones greatly, which means that you have a lot of great options to choose from. First, let's start with the best and easiest fruits and vegetables to work with. Apart from being easy to juice (depending on your juicer), these options will give you juice with a lovely flavor, especially when you find the right combinations of ingredients that complement each other well.

The Best Vegetables to Juice

Although pure vegetable juice isn't a very popular choice, especially among beginners, you can always start with juice blends that contain juice extracted from these healthy options. As you get used to juicing, then you can start experimenting with fresh vegetable juices to see which ones are palatable for you. The best and healthiest types of vegetables to juice are:

- **Beets**

   Beets have an earthy flavor and they offer a number of health benefits to your juice blends too. They contain folate, potassium, manganese, and nitrates. You can juice the root and even the leafy tops of beets to add to your juice blends. Either way, beets will add a boost of nutrition to your fresh beverages.

- **Broccoli**

   Broccoli is a rich source of potassium, vitamin A, and other essential micronutrients. This cruciferous vegetable also contains a powerful compound known as kaempferol that helps neutralize the effects of free radicals, reduce the growth of cancer cells, and decrease inflammation. You can add all parts of this vegetable in your juicer to add nutrition to your fresh juices.

- **Cabbage**

Although a glass of cabbage juice might not sound very appealing, this is still considered as one of the best veggies to juice. This is a nutritious vegetable that has a good flavor to complement other ingredients. Cabbage contains vitamin C, vitamin K, and a host of micronutrients. Since this is a cruciferous veggie, it offers a lot of health benefits making it another amazing choice.

- **Carrots**

Carrots have a lovely sweet flavor along with a healthy nutrient profile making them one of the best veggies to juice. This is a low-calorie vegetable that contains potassium, vitamin A, antioxidants, biotin, and other nutrients. If you want to make pure vegetable juice blends, adding carrots can provide a sweet taste to make the juice blends more palatable.

- **Celery**

These days, celery juice is all the rage. This vegetable is high in water, it contains different vitamins, and it's rich in antioxidants too. This veggie offers a number of health benefits, especially in terms of preventing the risk of chronic disease. While you can drink celery juice on its own, it also works well as an ingredient in juice blends.

- **Cucumbers**

Since cucumbers have a very high water content, this makes them an amazing veggie to juice. This is a low-calorie vegetable that contains manganese, potassium, and different types of vitamins. One of the best benefits of cucumbers is that it can help you stay hydrated. This is very important, especially when you are doing juice cleanses.

- **Kale**

Kale is a versatile vegetable that you can mix with other ingredients because of its mild flavor. When uncooked, kale is high in beta-carotene and other healthy antioxidants. It also contains vitamin A, vitamin C, vitamin K, and other essential nutrients to improve your health. Because of the many nutrients this veggie has to offer, it can help prevent the development of various diseases. It also protects the body against damages caused by free radicals.

- **Parsley**

Although you might not think of this herb as a healthy ingredient, it offers several health benefits too. It's not just a great garnish, it's also an excellent option for juicing. Parsley is rich in vitamin A, vitamin C, and vitamin K, among other nutrients. It also contains a lot of antioxidants to protect your body and keep you healthy.

- **Spinach**

When you think about leafy, green veggies, your mind would immediately go to spinach because this is one of the healthiest types. Spinach has a fresh, subtle flavor making it a perfect addition to fresh juices. It is high in antioxidants, vitamin C, vitamin A, and nitrates. If you suffer from acid reflux, adding this vegetable to your juicing regimen will be especially beneficial as it offers significant antacid benefits.

- **Swiss Chard**

Swiss chard is a leafy, green veggie that is chock-full of essential minerals, vitamins, and antioxidants. Adding this veggie in your juice will help you combat cellular damage more effectively. This vegetable is especially beneficial if you suffer from diabetes as it helps stabilize blood sugar levels.

- **Tomatoes**

This is another juicy veggie that's low-calorie but high in essential nutrients. In particular, tomatoes are high in lycopene that can reduce your risk of developing a number of diseases including cancer. Tomatoes have anti-inflammatory properties and they can even increase your metabolism.

- **Wheatgrass**

Wheatgrass is one of the more popular vegetables people use for juicing. It is a nutrient-dense veggie that's rich in copper, iron, magnesium, phosphorus, and several amino acids. Wheatgrass also contains chlorophyll which has potent cancer-fighting and anti-inflammatory properties. Whether drunk on its own or mixed in juice blends, this is an incredible choice for you.

Aside from these, other great options include basil, chard, cilantro, fennel, ginger root, mint, romaine lettuce, and sweet potato. Mix and match the veggies you use to create interesting combinations. If you're not a fan of veggies, you might become fond of these healthy food items when you start experiencing all of the health benefits they have to offer.

The Best Fruits to Juice

Juicing wouldn't be complete without fresh fruits. Although you should focus more on veggies when doing juice cleanses or supplementing your diet with juicing, fruits are a valuable addition because of their taste and because they are rich in nutrients too. Here are some of the best fruits for you to juice:

- **Apples**

    Apple juice is one of the most common types of juice you will find in stores. Apples are very healthy but if you want to get all of their healthy nutrients, it's best to juice fresh apples instead of buying processed apple juice products. This fruit is rich in antioxidants and it offers a lot of health benefits. Because of its sweet taste, apples make a great addition to juice blends too.

- **Berries**

    Berries are high in antioxidants and other nutrients making them another amazing choice for juicing. Some berries even offer antiviral and antibacterial properties. However, since berries are seasonal, you may have to work with what is available unless you want to spend more by purchasing berries that aren't in season. Of course, all berries are tasty and healthy so you can just include whatever's in season to your juices and still enjoy benefits to your health.

- **Citrus Fruits**

    Citrus fruits like oranges, lemons, and grapefruits are common juicing choices too. These fruits are very easy to juice, they always have a high yield, and they are chock-full of nutrients. Citrus fruits also have yummy flavors making them a great addition to your juice blends.

- **Papayas**

    Papayas are very beneficial, especially for your digestive health. This fruit contains papain, a type of enzyme that aids in protein breakdown. If you're having digestive or bowel issues, you may want to include this fruit in your juice blends or even have a glass of pure, fresh papaya juice once in a while.

When it comes to juicing, fruits are a lot easier and more appealing. Just remember that you are juicing for your health so try not to add too many fruits to ensure that your juice blends aren't too high in sugar. Aside from these, other great fruit options for juicing are cantaloupes, grapes, honeydew, kiwis, mangoes, peaches, pears, pineapples, plums, pomegranates, and watermelons. Try to mix and match these fruits and veggies to create interesting combinations. You can even add spices like cayenne pepper, ginger or paprika to make your juices more flavorful.

The Most Challenging Juicing Options

In general, the fruits and veggies that are challenging to juice are the ones that don't contain that much liquid. For some of these options, they produce a juice that isn't palatable at all. Here is a list for your reference:

Vegetables

- Eggplants
- Onions
- Rhubarb
- Sugar Cane

Fruits

- Avocadoes
- Bananas
- Coconuts
- Dried Fruits
- Figs
- Grains

- Winter Squash

While there are more options for fruits and vegetables that can be juiced easily, you may still have to watch what you juice, especially if you suffer from certain health issues. These include:

- **Blood Sugar Fluctuations**

    If you have issues with your blood sugar levels and you need to carefully manage these levels, then you should stay away from fruits with high sugar levels. You should also increase your veggie to fruit ratio when making juice blends. It's also recommended to speak with your doctor first before you start juicing.

- **Kidney Stones**

  If you have kidney stones or you have a history of kidney stones in the past, then you should avoid juicing fruits and veggies that are high in oxalates like bananas, chard, cherries, mangoes, and raw spinach, for example. Consumption of such foods in large amounts can either cause the formation of or worsen kidney stones.

- **Stomach Bloating**

  If you start juicing and you notice that you are always bloated afterward, then you may want to reduce or eliminate kale, bok choy, and other cruciferous veggies from your juice blends. Healthy and nutrient-dense as these veggies are, juicing them raw might be the reason why you experience stomach bloating. If you still want to include these veggies in your diet (and you should!), you may steam them lightly first before consumption.

- **Thyroid Problems**

  If you suffer from thyroid problems, you should also avoid raw cruciferous veggies as consuming too much of these might disrupt your thyroid functions. If you know that you have any type of thyroid issue, consult with your doctor first before juicing, especially if you want to include these veggies in your juice blends.

Of course, if you don't suffer from any kind of medical condition, you can juice different kinds of fruits, veggies, and fruit-veggie combinations. As long as you learn how to listen to your body to observe possible side effects, and deal with them, juicing can be a wonderful part of your life.

Finding the Best Juicing Recipes

Now that you know what to juice and what to avoid (or at least, minimize), the next thing to do is to plan your recipes. As a juicing beginner, you may start with simple juices and juice blends. Pure fruit juices and pure veggie juices are the easiest to make. Once you have gotten the hang of juicing and of using your juicer, then you can experiment with more complex recipes. By finding the right combinations of fruits and vegetables, you can create spectacular juices that taste great and will provide you with the nutrients you need to improve your health.

If this is your first juicing experience or if you are planning to do your first juice cleanse, it's recommended to plan your recipes. This will give you a chance to research the juices and juice blends to drink throughout your juice cleanse and how to prepare everything to make your juicing process more efficient. For instance, if your main health goal is to lose weight, then you can use ingredients that promote weight-loss. Or if you want to overcome certain health issues, choose ingredients that will help you achieve this. Here are some examples for you:

- Adding **cucumbers** to your juice blend promotes the health of your skin, lowers your blood pressure, and keeps you hydrated.
- Adding **ginger** to your juice blend helps reduce pain, improve your digestive system, and give your immune system a boost.
- Adding **green apples** to your juice blend helps lower cholesterol, increase your energy levels, and reduce inflammation.
- Adding **kale** to your juice blend provides anti-inflammatory and antioxidant properties to help you

overcome autoimmune diseases, arthritis, and even chronic disorders.

Juicing is such a versatile and customizable process, which is why it works so well. By doing your research, you can get all of the benefits juicing and juice cleanses have to offer. To help you plan your juice recipes better, here are some tips:

- Although sweet fruits are a wonderful addition to juice blends, great juice recipes aren't exclusively based on them. Other fruits and veggies also have lovely flavors and if you can find the right combinations, you can plan healthier recipes.

- When it comes to creating your own recipes, the optimal veggie to fruit ratio is 2:1. That way, you have all the goodness of vegetables with the tasty sweetness of fruits.

- Instead of always choosing sweet fruits to add flavor to your juice blends, why don't you give acidic fruits a try? These will make your juices taste great while adding nutrients to the mix.

- If you're not a fan of fruits or vegetables (especially the latter), you should try experimenting with ingredients that you don't usually incorporate in your diet. As long as you don't suffer from a medical condition that prevents you from consuming certain foods, then you can add as many veggies to your juices along with a few fruits to make things sweeter.

- Create a list of recipes along with a schedule for your juice cleanse. If you are interested in juicing to supplement your diet, then you can just keep a list of recipes to make each week. But if you are doing a juice cleanse, it's recommended to create a schedule too so that you will stay on track from the first day of your juice cleanse to the last.

Planning your juice recipes can be a lot of fun. As a beginner, you will learn how to find the healthiest juices, the most beneficial ingredients, and the best combinations. The longer you stay on your juicing journey, the more you will learn about what ingredients are easiest to prepare, which ingredients are in season, how different juices and juice blends affect you, and how to make your juicing processes as efficient as possible.

Preparing Your Juicing Ingredients

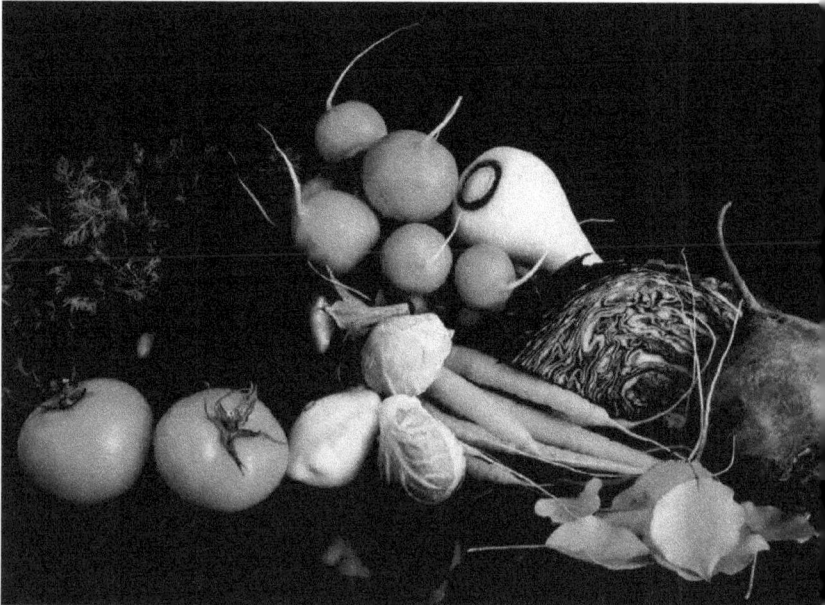

Fig. 6: Fresh Ingredients. Unsplash, by Sharon Pittaway, 2018,
https://unsplash.com/photos/KUZnfk-2DSQ/ Copyright 2018 by Sharon Pittaway/Unsplash

After planning your recipes, it's time to start preparing the produce for your juices. Go through your recipes and see which ingredients you need. Create a separate list of ingredients to bring with you to the supermarket so that you know exactly what you need. When it comes to choosing ingredients for juicing, it's best to opt for organic whenever possible.

Since you will be increasing your intake of fruits and veggies, you will also be increasing your risk of ingesting the pesticides used on the produce you buy. You can avoid this by going organic since organic produce typically contains fewer pesticides. Organic produce might be more expensive, but remember that you want to start juicing to improve your health. You can increase your chances of improving your health and reaching your health goals by going organic.

After purchasing your ingredients, decide whether you want to juice them raw or cook them first before juicing. When it comes to juicing, especially juice cleanses, it's more recommended to use the fruits and veggies in their raw form since cooking tends to kill or eliminate a lot of nutrients. And drinking juice made from raw fruits and veggies is healthier too since juice comes in liquid form, which is absorbed by the body easily. Before going through the best preparation methods of different fruits and veggies, here are some of the basic preparation tips for you:

- Whether you cook your ingredients or not, make sure to wash everything thoroughly before juicing. This is important even if you opt for organic ingredients to rinse off and hopefully, remove all traces of pesticides on the fruits and veggies.
- Even if your juicer has a large feeding chute, it's still recommended to peel, chop, and remove the seeds of fruits and veggies, especially if you don't want any pulp. This also makes it easier for your juicer to extract more liquid. But if the skin of the fruit or vegetable is edible and it won't change the taste of the juice, then you don't

have to peel it—just make sure you have washed it thoroughly.

Make sure to prepare your ingredients properly before juicing. Some fruits and veggies require more preparation than others. If you plan your recipes well, you can make complex juice recipes when you have a lot of time to prepare then opt for the easy-to-prep ingredients for when you don't have a lot of time like during the morning rush. To help you prepare your ingredients the right way, here are some tips for you:

Preparing Fruits

Fruits	Preparation Methods
Apples	Core the apples first and remove the seeds. You can also choose to slice the apples before juicing.
Apricots	After rinsing, slice the apricots in half, and remove the seed.
Avocados	For avocados, it's better to process them in a blender as you won't get a lot of juice from them. Cut the avocados in half, remove the pit, and spoon the flesh into your blender.
Bananas	For bananas, it's better to process them in a blender as you won't get a lot of juice from them. Peel the bananas first before adding to the blender.
Blackberries	Rinse the blackberries thoroughly then drain using a strainer. Do this right before juicing since blackberries don't keep well after you rinse them.
Blueberries	Rinse the blueberries thoroughly then drain using a strainer.
Cactus Pears	Peel the cactus pears first and chop them roughly before adding to your juicer.
Cantaloupe	Peel the cantaloupes, remove the seeds, and chop the flesh into chunks before adding to your juicer.

Cherries	Rinse the cherries well. With a paring knife, remove the pits before adding the cherries to your juicer. Add about a handful or more depending on the size of your juicer's feeding chute.
Cranberries	Rinse the cranberries well before adding to your juicer.
Grapefruit	Peel the grapefruits while trying to keep some of the white-colored pith as this part contains essential nutrients that aid with your body's absorption of antioxidants like vitamin C. After peeling, chop into chunks that fit into your juicer's feeding chute.
Grapes	Rinse the grapes well, pluck each grape from the stem, and remove the seeds before placing in your juicer.
Kiwi	Cut the kiwis in half and peel first before adding to your juicer.
Lemons	Peel the lemons while trying to keep some of the white-colored pith as this part contains essential nutrients that aid with your body's absorption of antioxidants like vitamin C. After peeling, chop into chunks that fit into your juicer's feeding chute. You may keep the seeds or leave them before juicing.
Limes	Peel the limes while trying to keep some of the white-colored pith as this part contains essential nutrients that aid with your body's absorption of

	antioxidants like vitamin C. After peeling, chop into chunks that fit into your juicer's feeding chute. You may keep the seeds or leave them before juicing.
Mangoes	Peel the mangoes and slice the flesh off of the pit before adding to your juicer.
Melons	Slice the melons into wedges then peel off the outer skin. Chop the wedges into smaller pieces. You may or may not remove the seeds before juicing.
Oranges	Peel the oranges while trying to keep some of the white-colored pith as this part contains essential nutrients that aid with your body's absorption of antioxidants like vitamin C. After peeling, chop into chunks that fit into your juicer's feeding chute. You may keep the seeds or leave them before juicing.
Papayas	Cut the papayas into quarters then peel the skin off. Then you can cut each quarter into smaller pieces before adding to your juicer. You may or may not remove the seeds before juicing.
Peaches	Slice the peaches in half and remove the pits before adding to your juicer.
Pears	First, rinse the pears thoroughly. If you have small pears, remove the stems, and juice them whole. For bigger pears, slice them first and remove the seeds before adding to your juicer.

Pineapples	Remove the entire top part of the pineapples. Slice the pineapples, remove the skin, and add t slices to your juicer. If needed, chop the pineapple slices into chunks to fit the feeding chute of your juicer.
Plums	Rinse the plums thoroughly first. Slice the plum in half and remove the pits before adding to you juicer.
Pomegranate	Prepare a bowl filled with water. Slice a pomegranate in half then submerge the whole fruit in water before breaking it apart. Use your hands to break the pomegranate into chunks the remove the seeds. After doing this, the white parts will float while the seeds will sink to the bottom of the bowl. With a slotted spoon, carefully take the seeds out and place them in your juicer.
Raspberries	Rinse the raspberries thoroughly then drain usin a strainer.
Strawberries	Rinse the strawberries thoroughly then drain using a strainer. Remove the stems before addin the strawberries to your juicer.
Sweet Potatoes	Scrub the sweet potatoes thoroughly to clean. Chop the sweet potatoes into chunks before adding to your juicer.

Tangerines	Peel the tangerines while trying to keep some of the white-colored pith as this part contains essential nutrients that aid with your body's absorption of antioxidants like vitamin C. After peeling, chop into chunks that fit into your juicer's feeding chute. You may keep the seeds or leave them before juicing.
Turnips	Scrub the turnips thoroughly to clean. Chop the turnips into chunks before adding to your juicer.
Watermelon	Slice the watermelons into wedges then peel off the rind and skin. Chop the wedges into smaller pieces. You may or may not remove the seeds before juicing.

Preparing Vegetables

Vegetables	Preparation Methods
Asparagus	Rinse the asparagus stalks thoroughly before adding to your juicer. When adding asparagus to the feeding chute, place the bottoms in first.
Beets	Peel the beets first and cut them into chunks before adding to your juicer. If you don't want to peel the beets, make sure to rinse and scrub them well before chopping, and adding to your juicer.
Bell Peppers	Rinse the bell peppers well. Remove the stems, cut in half, and add to your juicer. You don't have to remove the seeds.
Broccoli	Rinse the broccoli well, chop it into chunks, and add all of the parts into your juicer.
Butter Lettuce	Separate the leaves from one another and rinse them individually. Roll each leaf up before placing it in your juicer. It's recommended to juice a hard fruit or veggie after juicing butter lettuce (or any other leafy, green vegetable) to get the most juice.
Butternut Squash	Cut the butternut squash into quarters then peel the skin off. Since the skin of this vegetable is very tough, you may opt to keep the skin on. Then you can cut each quarter into smaller pieces before adding to your juicer. You may or may not remove the seeds before juicing.

Cabbage	Cut the head of cabbage into wedges that are small enough to fit into your juicer's feeding chute. When choosing cabbage heads, opt for those with crisp and firm leaves.
Carrots	Rinse the carrots thoroughly, chop into chunks, and add to your juicer. You may or may not peel carrots or remove the greens at the top before juicing.
Celery	Rinse the celery stalks thoroughly, chop into chunks, and add to your juicer, leaves, and all.
Celeriac	Rinse the celeriac thoroughly first to make sure that there aren't any grits left. Peel the celeriac and chop into chunks before adding to your juicer.
Chard	Separate the leaves from one another and rinse them individually. Roll each leaf up before placing it in your juicer. It's recommended to juice a hard fruit or veggie after juicing chard (or any other leafy, green vegetable) to get the most juice.
Cucumbers	Rinse the cucumbers, chop into chunks, and add to your juicer. You may or may not peel the cucumbers first before juicing.
Fennel Bulbs	Rinse the fennel bulbs thoroughly, chop into chunks, and add to your juicer.
Jalapeño	Rinse the jalapeño, remove the stem, and add to your juicer. Just remember that jalapeños are quite spicy so add them with care.

Jicama	Rinse the jicama thoroughly and chop into chunks before adding to your juicer. You don't have to peel it since the skin contains a lot of nutrients.
Kale	Separate the leaves from one another and rinse them individually. Roll each leaf up before placir it in your juicer. It's recommended to juice a har fruit or veggie after juicing kale (or any other leafy, green vegetable) to get the most juice.
Leeks	Slice the leeks in half lengthwise without removing the green parts or the roots. Separate the layers carefully while rinsing without detaching the layers from one another. If needec slice the leeks into smaller pieces to fit the feedir chute of your juicer.
Mustard Greens	Separate the leaves from one another and rinse them individually. Roll each leaf up before placir it in your juicer. It's recommended to juice a har fruit or veggie after juicing mustard greens (or ar other leafy, green vegetable) to get the most juic But for this vegetable, don't use too many leaves as mustard greens have a very potent flavor.
Onions	This is another veggie that you shouldn't add too much of since onions have a strong flavor. Peel off the skin of the onions and slice before addin to your juicer.
Parsnips	Rinse the parsnips thoroughly, chop into chunks and add to your juicer. You may or may not peel

	parsnips or remove the greens at the top before juicing.
Radishes	Rinse the radishes thoroughly, chop into chunks, and add to your juicer. You may or may not peel parsnips or remove the roots before juicing. But you should remove the leaves before adding the radishes to your juicer. Also, you shouldn't add too many radishes since they have a strong flavor.
Romaine Lettuce	Separate the leaves from one another and rinse them individually. Roll each leaf up before placing it in your juicer. It's recommended to juice a hard fruit or veggie after juicing romaine lettuce (or any other leafy, green vegetable) to get the most juice.
Scallions	Rinse the scallions thoroughly before adding to your juicer. This veggie has a strong flavor too, so add small amounts at a time.
Spinach	Rinse spinach well to remove all the grit. Roll bunches of leaves into a ball before adding to your juicer. It's recommended to juice a hard fruit or veggie after juicing romaine lettuce (or any other leafy, green vegetable) to get the most juice.
Squashes	Cut the squash into quarters then peel the skin off. Since the skin of this vegetable is very tough, you may opt to keep the skin on. Then you can cut each quarter into smaller pieces before adding to your juicer. You may or may not remove the seeds before juicing.

Sugar Snap Peas	Rinse the sugar snap peas before adding to your juicer. However, this veggie doesn't contain a lot of water so you should juice it along with other veggies and fruits.
Tomatoes	Rinse the tomatoes thoroughly, remove the stem and leaves, then add to your juicer. If you have big tomatoes, slice them first. You don't have to remove the seeds.
Wheatgrass	Rinse the wheatgrass thoroughly. Roll the wheatgrass into a ball or twist it then add to the feeding chute of your juicer. Just like leafy, green veggies, it's recommended to juice a hard fruit or veggie after juicing wheatgrass to get the most juice.
Zucchinis	Rinse the zucchinis well, cut the stem off, and chop into chunks before adding to your juicer.

Herbs and Spices

Herbs and spices can also be part of your juices and juice blends. You can add some of these to your juicer while adding others directly to the extracted juice. Here is a quick guide for you:

- For **basil**, rinse the leaves thoroughly to remove all grit. Roll the basil leaves into balls before adding into your juicer.
- For **cilantro**, wash thoroughly before adding the leaves and stems to your juicer.
- For **cinnamon**, use ground cinnamon and sprinkle over the juice directly.
- For **dill**, rinse thoroughly then gently pull off the fronds from the stem before juicing.
- For **garlic**, peel it first before adding to your juicer. Just remember that garlic has a strong flavor so don't add too much.
- For **ginger**, peel the ginger first before adding to your juicer.
- For **mint**, rinse it thoroughly first then remove the leaves before juicing.
- For **parsley**, rinse the leaves carefully to remove the grits. Tear the leaves off then roll into balls before adding into your juicer.
- For **tarragon**, rinse it thoroughly then tear the leaves off then roll into balls before adding into your juicer.

When it comes to cleaning up, one of the messiest parts is the pulp that gets left behind. No matter how efficient your juicer is, it might still produce a lot of solid waste depending on the ingredients you use. If you want to make cleanup an easier task, use a sheet of plastic wrap to line your juicer's pulp collection bin.

After juicing, simply remove the plastic wrap along with the waste.

The Aftermath of Juicing

Juicing doesn't have to be a complicated process. In fact, if you have a powerful juicer, you hardly need to make any preparations—mostly rinsing. Remember that juices are best consumed when fresh. If you want to get the most health benefits and the best taste, drink your juice right after extraction. But with the right juicer, you can store the juices you make in an airtight container then place them in your refrigerator. This is the next best thing if you don't have time to prep your ingredients each time. Another option is to make big batches of juice and pour them in mason jars. Then place the jars in your freezer until you're ready to drink them. But if you do this, make sure to leave space on top as juice tends to expand when you freeze them. If not, your mason jars might explode in the freezer!

One of the best parts of juicing is to drink freshly-made juice. It's even better if you have new recipes or it's the first time for you to try fresh fruit or veggie juice. Since juicing doesn't involve cooking (ideally), you don't have to learn special techniques. If you juice regularly, you will become very fast and very efficient at prepping ingredients. After extracting all the healthy goodness of juice, what comes next? What do you do with the peels and pulp when you're done juicing? Do you just throw it all away?

Not necessarily.

Although most people would simply throw away these "solid waste," you don't have to, especially when you consider how nutrient-dense the pulp and peels are. This means that they can also provide your body with health benefits. With a powerful juicer, you won't have to peel the fruits or veggies before juicing them. But if your juicer cannot handle hard fruits and veggies well, make sure to peel your produce before juicing, especially ingredients with thick rinds like pineapples or squash. You don't want to clog your juicer. But whether you peel the fruits and veggies or not, you will always be left with some byproducts that you might wonder what to do with. Fortunately, the aftermath of juicing doesn't always have to end up in the trash. You can do so many things with peels, pulp, and even seeds! Here are some ideas for you:

Smoothies

Once in a while, you can create smoothies instead of juices. For this, you need a blender. When blending fruits and veggies, you can include the peels and pulp since blenders are powerful enough to process these parts of produce. Adding pulp will make your smoothies thicker to give you a milk-shake consistency. Pulp and peels will also add fiber to your smoothies making them more satisfying. Although you won't taste these while drinking your smoothies, your body will get all of the nutrients they contain.

Broth

Have you ever tried making broth? All you have to do is boil bones for hours to get a flavorful broth that's rich in nutrients. Adding the leftover pulp from the veggies you juice will make your broth tastier and healthier too.

Healthy Recipes

If you enjoy cooking, you can work the unused parts of the fruits and veggies into healthy recipes for dips, sauces, and desserts, for example. These will give your recipes an interesting texture and flavor while adding a nutrient boost too.

Baked Goods

Just as you can add the pulp to healthy recipes, you can add fruit and veggie pulp to baked goods too. From muffins to loaves, and more, you can make your baked creations healthier by adding these ingredients. They might even make your baked goods taste better.

Scrambled Eggs

Do you enjoy eggs for breakfast? Then why don't you add your leftover vegetable pulp to your eggs? This will give you a scrumptious, nutrient-filled breakfast.

Flavored Ice Cubes

This is a fun and yummy way to use your juicing leftovers. Add them to a tray of ice cubes with water, and freeze them. Then you can add these flavored ice cubes to a glass of water for a more refreshing, flavorful, and healthy beverage.

Composting

If you don't want to consume these parts at all, don't throw them away just yet! Instead, use them as compost for your plants. If you have a garden, you can place the solid waste you get from juicing here. If you will be juicing regularly, you can expect your plants to thrive and bloom too.

Try to be as creative as possible when using your juicing leftovers. This will allow you to reduce your food waste significantly. Experiment. Have fun. You might even discover some amazing combinations that you will enjoy. A large part of juicing is discovering new things. You will learn all the basics in this eBook but when you start juicing, you will discover a lot more. For instance, there are certain mistakes that you have to avoid while juicing. Here are the most common ones:

- When you make the same type of juice blend over and over again, you will get bored. Even if you find a combination or a type of juice that you really love, if you drink it every day, you will eventually get tired of it. Also, your body needs different nutrients and enzymes. You can only get all of these by varying your juices and juice blends.

- If you don't wash your produce well, you might end up getting sick. Whether you choose organic fruits and veggies or not, any leftover dirt, pesticides, and grit will be going into your juice too. Rinsing and scrubbing are the most important steps in your prepping process, so don't skip them.

- If you don't listen to your body, you won't know what works for you and what doesn't. While juicing, you should observe how your body reacts to different juices. Even your timings should be observed carefully. If you want juicing to improve your health, listening to your body is key.

By knowing all of the basics of juicing, you can start planning to achieve your goals. You may want to lose weight, overcome an illness or simply improve your health. No matter what your health goals are, creating a plan will help make things easier for you, especially when it comes to juicing.

Chapter 4:

Juicing for Weight Loss

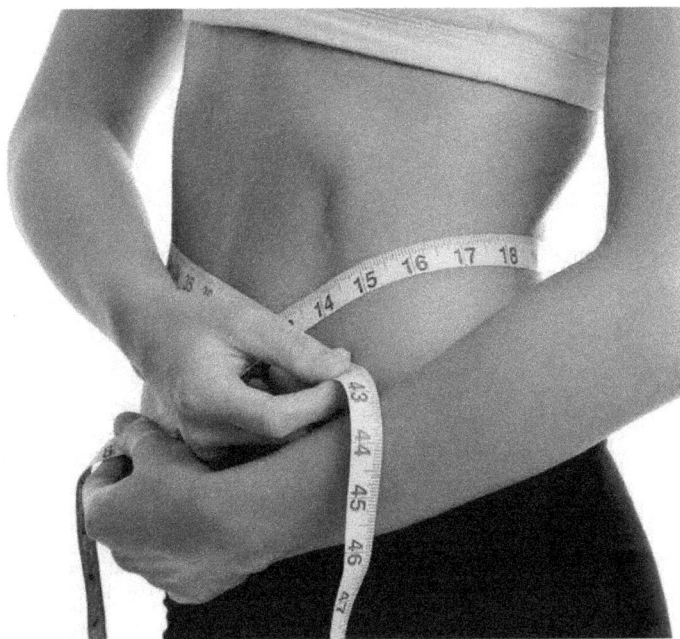

Most people who become interested in juicing want to detoxify their bodies and lose weight. These are the most common reasons why people, myself included, choose to start juicing. Then you realize that this healthy habit comes with more health benefits that you bargained for! When you drink nutrient-dense juice made from fresh fruits and vegetables, you can't go wrong! And if weight loss is your main health goal, juicing will definitely help you achieve this.

You can juice your fruits and veggies by hand but if you want juicing to be a regular part of your life or you plan to do juice cleanses regularly, especially to lose weight, then you should consider investing in a juicer that fits into your budget. Then you can juice to your heart's content and make healthy, tasty juices that promote weight loss. In this chapter, we will be focusing on the weight loss benefit of juicing. Here, you will learn why juicing can help you lose weight, how you can get the most out of this benefit, and so much more.

How Juicing Can Help You Lose Weight

Supplementing your diet with fresh juice and doing regular juice cleanses are great ways to kick-start your weight-loss journey. However, you should always remember that juices should not be used to replace your meals. If you do this, you will definitely lose weight. But restricting yourself severely in this way might change the way your body works and the worst thing that can happen is your metabolism slows down. When this happens, you will regain all of the weight you have lost, and then some, when you go back to eating full meals.

If you want to lose weight, one of the most effective things you can do is to reduce your daily caloric intake. You can drink a fresh glass of juice before your meals to make you feel fuller, but don't drink juice only for your meals. Since doing this will make you feel full, you will end up eating smaller portions. And if you do this regularly while still maintaining a healthy, balanced diet, you will notice yourself shedding those stubborn excess pounds without compromising your health in the process. Juicing should be part of your life—not just a quick fix for you to reach your weight loss goals in a short amount of time.

While there isn't a lot of formal research and studies that support the weight loss benefit of juicing, there is more than enough anecdotal evidence out there. As you already know, I am one of those people who has successfully lost weight because of juicing, and until now, I still drink juice regularly. By learning how to use juicing properly, you can make it sustainable and beneficial. But if you start experiencing adverse side effects because of juicing, you should either stop or modify your strategies until you experience benefits instead of adverse effects.

To achieve weight loss through juicing, it's all about using the right strategies. For instance, there are specific ingredients and recipes you can use to stimulate a fat-burning or 'thermogenic' effect for effective weight loss. Pair these juices with a healthy, balanced diet, and regular exercise to help you reach your goals.

Embracing Greens

If losing weight and burning fat are your main goals, then you should focus more on veggies while juicing. The key to making juice blends that promote weight loss is embracing your greens. Do this by creating juice blends that contain green veggies as the bulk of the mixture. Green juices are rich in nutrients like chlorophyll, a compound found in plants that aids in the oxygenation of the body. This will help cleanse and detoxify your body, improve blood circulation, and increase your energy levels, all of which may help in weight loss.

Juicing for weight loss means finding the right ingredients to promote this benefit. Since juices are easily absorbed by the body, drinking juices that are mainly composed of veggies would be like giving yourself a shot of enzymes, vitamins, and minerals in one go. However, if you focus too much on fruits because you want your juices to taste sweet, then you might not achieve the results you're hoping for. Although green juices may take some getting used to, you will surely feel motivated once you notice yourself losing weight. Aside from weight loss, adding more greens to your juices offer the following benefits too:

Veggies Contain High Levels of Nutrients

Vegetables are more nutrient-dense compared to fruits and they seldom contain sugar too. Therefore, drinking a glass of veggie juice or at least, a glass of juice that mainly contains vegetables will provide your body with a lot of essential antioxidants and nutrients. If you can combine different vegetables in a single juice blend, that would be even better! You will be consuming all of the nutrients of the individual vegetables in liquid form, which your body absorbs easily.

Veggies Promote Nutrient Absorption

Although you should be eating a lot of veggies, it takes time for your body to break these down to absorb all of the nutrients. In juice form, your body gains easy access to those nutrients almost immediately. You don't even have to worry about your body not being able to process the veggies because you didn't chew them properly. Your juicer would have already extracted most of the nutrients from the veggies and all your body has to do is absorb all of the healthy goodness.

Veggies Keep You Hydrated

Drinking enough water throughout the day is important to stay strong and healthy. But if you want to make sure that you never get dehydrated, drink fresh vegetable juice at different times of the day. Aside from all of the nutrients, fresh vegetable juices also contain water to make you feel hydrated, rejuvenated, and active throughout the day.

Veggies Promote the Health of Your Hair

Apart from helping you lose weight, vegetable juices can also give you healthier hair. For this benefit, make sure to include spinach, onions, carrots, and beetroots to your juices to revitalize your locks and promote healthy hair growth. Green juices can even combat hair loss, especially peppers and cauliflower. While you're losing weight, try to observe your hair too. You might be surprised at how much it improves.

Veggies Promote the Health of Your Skin

Your hair isn't the only one that will improve. You will also start noticing improvements in your skin too. For one, adding carrots, pumpkins, and sweet potatoes to your juices will help cure pimples and acne. Orange-colored veggies and those rich in vitamin C will provide you with this benefit too. If you want to have healthier, glowing skin, then you should add radishes, cabbages, tomatoes, and carrots to your juice blends. These will help your skin become radiant. And if you want to prevent or even treat wrinkles, opt for cauliflower, tomatoes, peppers, broccoli, and other veggies that contain high levels of vitamin C. Also, opt for vitamin E rich veggies like turnip greens and collard greens to keep these common signs of aging at bay.

If you learn how to embrace your veggies, weight loss won't be the only benefit to look forward to. Of course, you don't have to stay away from fruits completely. Just make sure that the bulk of your juices are veggies. Also, opt for fruits that can help promote weight loss while adding sweetness to your drinks.

Timing is the Key

When it comes to juicing for weight loss, proper timing is important. For instance, doing regular juice cleanses can help you lose weight while detoxifying your body. But if you're not on a cleanse that is completely juice-based, then you should drink a glass of juice around thirty minutes before having your meals. This will give your body hydration, a boost of nutrients, and it can make you feel full. That way, you won't feel like consuming large portions and you won't feel strong cravings either.

After some time, if you have fruit juice cravings, it's best to have juice in the morning too. This will give your body the energy it needs for the rest of the morning. Since fruit juice contains sugar, your body will be able to use that sugar throughout the day. Another great benefit of drinking juice first thing in the morning is that it helps eliminate any food residue from the day before. Drinking your juice at this time of the day cleanses your digestive tract and stomach, enabling your body to absorb nutrients fully.

Another great timing for drinking juice is in the afternoon. As your body begins winding down and you start getting tired, drinking a glass of fresh juice gives you energy too. Juice will give you a nutrient boost, provide more hydration, and increase your energy levels until the evening right before you go to sleep.

Although you shouldn't drink juice as a replacement for your meals, it's better to drink juice on an empty stomach. This will allow your body to absorb all of the healthy nutrients in the juice as it won't be bust breaking down solid foods. Since juice comes in liquid form, your digestive processes won't have to do much work. Despite this, you will still be giving your body a boost of nutrition to ensure optimal health. As time goes by, you will start noticing the wonderful changes in your body.

While there are perfect timings for drinking your juice, there are also timings that you should avoid while juicing. For one, you shouldn't wait for a long time before drinking your freshly-made juice. Leaving your glass of juice on the counter for a long time would be like robbing yourself of the many nutrients you should have received from the juice. Typically, after about 15 minutes, air and light will start having a deteriorating effect on many of the nutrients in your juice. Aside from this, the antioxidant content of your juice will also start losing its potency.

Then there is the amount of time you drink your juice. Fresh juice isn't meant to be consumed in a matter of seconds like shots of alcohol. Instead, you should take the time to sit down and enjoy your juice until you finish it. You can even drink mouthfuls of juice and swirl the juice in your mouth before you swallow it. Doing this stimulates your digestive enzymes to make it even easier for your body to process the juice that you are drinking. If you don't have time to drink your juice luxuriously, just try not to gulp it down in a matter of seconds.

All About Juice Fasting

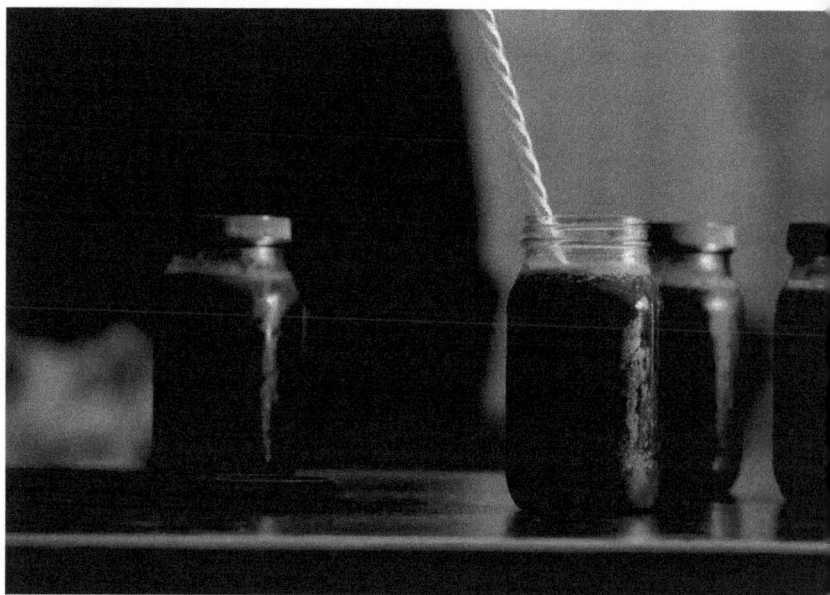

Fig. 8: Juice Cleanses. Unsplash, by K15 Photos, 2019, https://unsplash.com/photos/VOdONjAP_Lk/ Copyright 2019 by K15 Photos/Unsplash.

Juicing isn't a single process or diet that you must follow. In fact, it is highly customizable depending on your preferences, and health goals. One of the most common juicing methods is a juice cleanse or a juice fast. This involves replacing your meals with fresh fruit and vegetable juices for a certain number of days. The last part is very important—you should only do this for a set number of days, not long-term.

There are many reasons why people do juice cleanses, one of which is to lose weight. Juice cleanses or juice fasts can help you lose weight because you will be abstaining from the consumption of solid food. However, you will still be consuming a lot of nutrients through the juices that you drink. A juice cleanse is very different from juicing for the purpose of supplementation. If you only plan to supplement your diet through juicing, then you can do this long-term.

Aside from helping you lose weight, juice cleanses do wonders for the body because of their detoxification benefit. As you drink fresh juice during your juice cleanse, you will be supplying your body with vitamins, minerals, nutrients, and organic water to wash out toxins and replenish your nutrients. For your first few juice cleanses, you may eat light snacks if you really feel hungry. Just make sure to avoid alcohol, animal products, bread, grains, and any form of sugar. The more you practice juice cleanses, the more you will learn how to survive for a number of days without eating any solids. Of course, weight loss and detoxification aren't the only benefits of doing juice cleanses. Apart from the general benefits of juicing, juice cleanses can provide the following benefits too:

- An improvement in your appetite, mood, and energy levels, especially after the juice cleanse.
- An improvement in your body's ability to absorb nutrients, which allows you to benefit from the nutrients the juices contain.
- A reduction of your caloric intake along with an increase in your nutrient intake.

Typically, juice cleanses result in weight loss, although only short-term. After your juice cleanse, you will stop losing weight. If you continue supplementing your healthy, balanced diet with juicing, you may continue losing weight but at a much slower pace. However, if you stop juicing and you go back to your high-calorie diet, then you might regain all of the weight that you have lost. Another reason why it's not recommended to extend juice cleanses for long periods of time is that you will be depriving yourself of solid foods for too long. When you go back to your normal diet, there is a very high likelihood that you will overindulge and overeat. Naturally, this will cause you to gain more weight, which is the exact opposite of your goals. Do juice cleanses once in a while but always go back to a healthy, balanced diet supplemented with juicing.

Now, the next question you must have is: how long should your juice cleanse be? The answer to this is up to you. As a beginner, you can try doing juice cleanses for only one or two days. After getting used to only drinking juice throughout the day, you can increase your juice cleanse to three or four days. If you have become a juice cleanse master, then you may do a cleanse for one whole week—but only after doing a couple of shorter juice cleanses. Apart from the juice cleanse itself, you need to have three to five days to prepare your body for the juice cleanse. Three to five days where you would eliminate foods from your diet gradually (before the juice cleanse) and three to five days where you would gradually reintroduce foods into your system. These pre- and post-cleansing days are very important to avoid the potential adverse side effects of juice cleanses.

One thing I can say to you about juice cleanses is that they are not as easy as they seem. Prepare yourself for a lot of new experiences like cravings, hunger, and frustration, for example. This is why it's important to plan for your juice cleanses from the juices you will drink, the schedule you will follow, and even the activities that you will do during your juice cleanse. As a beginner, you should start slow so that you won't end up causing stress to your body or mind.

Right now, there isn't enough research that shows how juice cleanses can help you lose weight in the long-term. However, the short-term results you will see will surely motivate you while kick-starting your weight loss process. Just make sure to do the juice cleanse properly so that you enjoy all of the benefits instead of experiencing the adverse side effects. When you're done with your juice cleanse, continue following a healthy diet to ensure that you continue losing weight. The best thing about juicing is that you are adding nutrients to your body without adding too many calories to your diet. Therefore, even if you lose weight, you will still remain healthy thanks to the nutrients in the juices that you drink.

Preparing Yourself for Juice Fasting

Although there aren't any standard rules to follow for a juice cleanse, there is a right way to do it, and a wrong way. The right way to do a juice cleanse ensures that you gain all the benefits of the cleanse without compromising your health in any way. The wrong way may cause you to experience adverse side effects or worse, long-term consequences to your health. To do a juice cleanse the right way involves preparing your body for it first.

Before you do your juice cleanse, you must take a few days to prepare your mind and body for it. Starting a juice cleanse right away can be very dangerous, especially if you are currently following a very unhealthy or unbalanced diet. After only a few hours, you might get sick or you might experience the adverse side effects of juice cleanses. To prepare yourself for your first juice cleanse, you should first transition to a healthier, more balanced diet. As you transition, you can also start juicing to supplement your diet. By supplementing your diet, you can get a hang of juicing from preparing the ingredients, experimenting with recipes, and getting used to the effects of different juices. This will make it easier for you to follow through with your juice cleanses.

As you prepare yourself for your juice cleanse, start increasing the vegetable content of your juice blends. Remember that juicing should focus more on veggies instead of fruits. If you plan to drink nothing but fruit juice on the days when you do your juice cleanse, you won't experience the benefits you are looking for. Fruits contain a lot of sugar, which doesn't make them the ideal option for your juices. At most, you should only add around one or two fruits to your juice blend to make it taste sweet while adding more nutrients to it. If weight loss is one of your goals, make sure to choose fruits that promote weight loss too. Then you can make your juices more flavorful by adding herbs and spices depending on your preferences.

It's better to experiment with juices and juice blends before you start your juice cleanse so that you can include your favorite juices in your plan. Then when it's time for you to start your juice cleanse, you can enjoy all of your favorite juices to make the whole process easier, more enjoyable, and less intimidating. Once in a while, you can also make smoothies for yourself. These are thicker, more filling, and more acceptable as a meal replacement, especially if you add a lot of ingredients to your smoothies. Even during your juice cleanse, you can have smoothies once in a while to fill you up and make you feel satisfied.

After preparing for your first juice cleanse, the next step is to create your plan for it. Create a plan for one to two days first and see how your body reacts to the juice cleanse. Your first cleanse shouldn't be longer than three days. Throughout the first day, observe your body carefully. You can even keep a journal where you note down which juices make you feel satisfied, which juices make you feel hungry right away, and which juices cause you adverse side effects. Writing these things down allows you to make a better, more effective plan for your next juice cleanse.

Creating Your Juice Cleanse Schedule

After preparing yourself for your first juice cleanse, it's time to think about your schedule. You can come up with a schedule well before the cleanse or you can create one while in the pre-cleanse stage. The length of this stage depends on your current diet and lifestyle. If you are following a healthy, balanced diet, then you may only set aside a couple of days for your pre-cleanse. But if you start with an unhealthy diet that's rich in processed, fast or junk foods, then you may have to transition to a healthier diet then have a longer pre-cleanse stage—at least four to seven days. While preparing, you should also drink a lot of water to ensure that you are always well hydrated. To help you create your juice cleanse schedule, here are some tips:

- Create a schedule with timings and the type of juice or juice blend you will drink. Include the name of the recipe so that you can easily refer to your recipe book when it's time for you to drink your juices.

- You should be drinking one glass of juice every 1 to 2 1/2 hours. The frequency depends on the type of juice you drink. For instance, if you drink a heavy smoothie for lunch, then you can have your next glass of juice after 2 1/2 hours. But if you have a light juice blend for breakfast, then you may have your next glass of juice after an hour. You can use your schedule to guide you.

- Make sure to remain consistent throughout your juice cleanse. While creating your schedule, you might think that drinking around six to eight glasses of juices throughout the day is a lot. But remember that you will only be consuming these juices and nothing else. So make sure that your schedule allows you to drink all the juice you need to have enough energy to get through the day.

When it's time for you to follow your schedule, make sure to follow it as closely as possible. For instance, try not to skip your juicing schedules even if you're not feeling particularly hungry yet. Since you will only be drinking liquids, your body needs each glass of juice to stay healthy and hydrated. Don't forget to include the post-juicing stage in your schedule. This happens after your juice cleanse and it involves gradually introducing solid food back into your diet. The type of juice cleanse you want to do can also have an effect on your schedule. Also, the type of juice cleanse you do will help you determine the types of juices that you will drink. Here are some examples:

- **Advanced Juice Cleanse**

  It's recommended to try this juice cleanse after you have experienced some simpler juice cleanses. This involves low-glycemic fruits and veggies making it perfect if you're following a low-sugar diet or you want to experience a deeper detoxification process.

- **Basic Juice Cleanse**

  Whether you are a beginner or an experienced juice cleanser, you can do this type of cleanse. Here, you would drink juice blends that contain fruits rich in minerals combined with alkaline veggies that are rich in antioxidants.

- **Rejuvenating Juice Cleanse**

  For this juice cleanse, you will combine freshly made juices with healthy broths, soups, and even superfoods for your snacks. This isn't a complete juice cleanse but it will make you feel rejuvenated. If you're a beginner, you may try this juice cleanse first.

Of course, you can also create your own type of juice cleanse along with your own schedule. Customizing your own juice cleanse makes it easier for you to follow your schedule while staying motivated until the end.

Chapter 5:

The Best Juicing Recipes for

Weight Loss

If your main goal for juicing is to lose weight, then you must learn how to choose the right ingredients and ingredient combinations to help you reach your goal. While weight loss is one of the main benefits of juicing, you should also make wise choices if you want to make the most out of this benefit. In this chapter, we will go through different types of pure juices and juice combinations that you may want to focus on to promote weight loss while juicing.

Pomegranate Juice

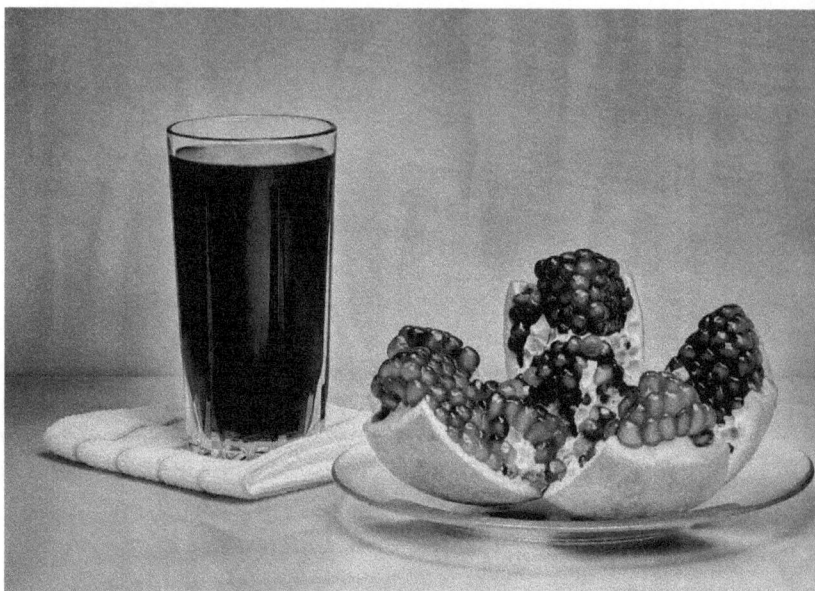

Fig. 9: Pomegranate Juice. Pixabay, by Michael Tavrionov, 2019,
https://pixabay.com/photos/pomegranate-juice-vitamin-red-3977500/ Copyright 2019 by
Michael Tavrionov/Pixabay.

Pomegranate juice is sweet, healthy, and an excellent option for when you're juicing to lose weight. The reason for this beneficial effect is that pomegranates contain high levels of conjugated linolenic acid, antioxidants, and polyphenols. All of these compounds help give your metabolism a boost while promoting the fat-burning process. Also, pomegranate juice can help suppress your appetite. Naturally, if you don't feel hungry, you won't feel the need to eat.

Drinking fresh pomegranate juice that you have made from fresh pomegranates is healthier and more refreshing than processed drinks that are typically laden with added sugar. As a bonus, pomegranate juice won't just help you lose weight. It also promotes healthy skin so you may notice your skin going back to your natural glow as you keep drinking this fresh beverage. You can make fresh pomegranate juice in your juicer by following these simple steps:

- Cut a fresh pomegranate in half, crosswise.
- Lift the handle of your juicer and place one half of the pomegranate on it with the fleshy part facing down.
- Press down using moderate pressure and watch as fresh juice flows out of the fruit. Continue pressing until you feel like you have extracted all the juice from the fruit.
- Keep juicing pomegranate halves until you have enough juice for one glass.
- If you want pure juice without seeds, you can pass it through a strainer first.

If the pomegranate fruit that you have juiced isn't sweet enough, you may add a natural sweetener to your juice. But if your main goal is to lose weight, then you may have to train yourself to enjoy fresh fruit juices without adding any sugar. It might be a bit difficult when you're first starting out but once you get used to the taste of fresh juice, you will learn to enjoy it.

Watermelon Juice

Watermelon is one of the easiest fruits to juice mainly because it mainly consists of water. This fruit will keep you hydrated at a mere 30 calories for every 100 grams that you drink. Although it is one of the sweeter fruits, it can still help promote weight loss. Watermelon contains high levels of arginine, an amino acid that promotes fat-burning. This fruit is also rich in other nutrients making it perfect for weight loss, cleansing, and fasting. It also provides you with electrolytes to help balance your body's electrolyte levels. Watermelon offers protein, fiber, and virtually no fat and cholesterol.

The great thing about watermelon juice is that it's thirst-quenching and refreshingly-sweet. Since it also offers nutritional benefits, you may want to stock up on watermelons to make fresh juice with your juicer. Here are the steps to do this:

- Cut the watermelon in half then continue cutting the fruit into cubes.
- Remove the seeds from the flesh. You may leave the white, tender seeds if you don't mind a bit of texture in your juice.
- Place the watermelon cubes in your juicer then press down to get fresh juice flowing. Continue juicing watermelon cubes until you have enough for one glass.

Watermelon juice contains phytonutrients, minerals, and vitamins. This juice also offers anti-inflammatory benefits from its triterpenoid and lycopene content. So if you're making a juicing schedule or plan, don't forget to add pure watermelon juice to help you shed excess pounds on your juice cleanse.

Grapefruit Juice

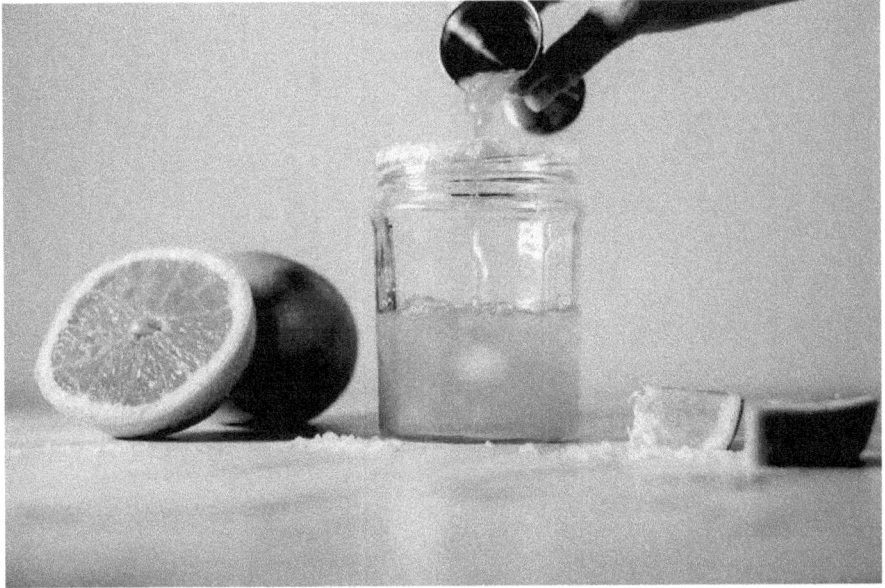

Fig. 10: Grapefruit Juice. Unsplash, by Rinck Content Studio, 2019, https://unsplash.com/photos/4pJekgmSmPM/ Copyright 2019 by Rinck Content Studio/Unsplash.

When you're trying to add fruits to your diet for the purpose of losing weight, grapefruit will always be at the top of the list. In fact, the grapefruit diet became very popular as a way to lose weight. While you won't be drinking grapefruit juice exclusively while juicing, fresh juice made from this fruit can help you lose weight while promoting your overall health. Drinking a glass of grapefruit juice helps improve your insulin resistance while curbing your appetite. Over time, these effects will make it easier for you to lose weight.

Personally, I have experienced the effects of drinking grapefruit juice in terms of weight loss. While preparing myself for a juice cleanse, I started drinking grapefruit juice right before eating my meals. This made me feel full and ultimately, I ended up eating smaller portions. Whether you are preparing for a juice cleanse or you're creating a plan for your 3-day or 7-day juice fast, grapefruit juice would be an excellent option. Here are some simple steps to make fresh grapefruit juice using your juicer:

- Rinse the grapefruit thoroughly using warm water.
- Cut the grapefruit in half, crosswise.
- Place one grapefruit half in your juicer with the fleshy side facing down.
- Press down on your juicer until fresh, pink juice starts flowing.
- Repeat these steps until you fill an entire glass with fresh juice.

By drinking grapefruit juice, you will boost your intake of vitamin C. This juice also contains dietary fiber, magnesium, and potassium. Combine this with a healthy, balanced diet, and regular exercise, and you're sure to start shedding those stubborn excess pounds. Of course, this is just one option that can help you lose weight. If you want to make juicing more sustainable for you, drinking a variety of weight-loss promoting juices is key.

Carrot Juice

When it comes to making fresh juice from veggies to promote weight loss, carrots are one of the best choices. Carrots are low in calories and fat but they are rich in nutrients. Juicing carrots is very healthy as the process makes it easier for your body to absorb the nutrients. Aside from being highly nutrient-dense, carrots also make you feel full for a longer time. This means that you won't crave for snacks as much, which is very helpful if you're on a juice cleanse.

Carrot juice is full of fiber, low in calories, and it's best if you have made the juice using raw carrots. It's best to drink this juice for breakfast to make you feel full right away. Carrot juice helps increase the secretion of bile, which helps your body burn fat. This is why it's a great option for weight loss. To make a glass of fresh carrot juice, here are some steps:

- Wash the carrots thoroughly using cold running water. If you have a vegetable brush, it's better to use it to clean the carrots better.
- Cut the broad end of the carrots with a knife.
- You may or may not peel the carrots. Either way, you won't be reducing the nutritional value significantly.
- Chop the carrots to make them easier to juice. But if you have a powerful juicer, you may skip this step.
- Place the carrot pieces in your juicer then press down until fresh juice starts flowing. Keep doing this until you have obtained one glass of fresh carrot juice.

Although it's best to enjoy carrot juice for breakfast, you can also drink it at any time. Carrots contain antioxidants too, which can help boost your immune system. This is an important benefit if you're trying to lose weight.

Cabbage Juice

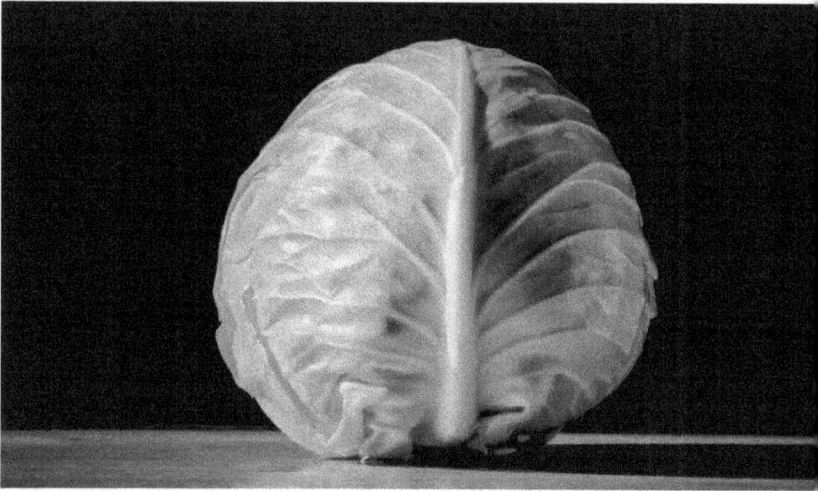

Fig. 11: Cabbage Juice. Unsplash, by C Drying, 2020,
https://unsplash.com/photos/BLV4pffJshA/ Copyright 2020 by C Drying/Unsplash.

Cabbage juice is an excellent choice for flushing out buildup in your digestive tract to optimize your digestive process. With a healthier digestive system, losing weight becomes easier. Fresh cabbage juice relieves issues like indigestion, bloating, and it helps you eliminate waste more efficiently. These effects also help with the process of weight loss. Another weight-loss benefit of cabbage is that it contains a lot of fiber, which can help your body combat fat.

High-fiber veggies like cabbage slow the process of digestion down so that you feel full for a longer time. Although fresh cabbage juice isn't the best-tasting type of juice, you can combine this with fruits like apple or beetroot to make it taste better. But if you're interested in making pure cabbage juice, you can follow these steps:

- Choose a head of cabbage that is firm and has crisp leaves. This type of cabbage will produce more juice compared to heads of cabbage with limp, yellowing leaves.
- Rinse the cabbage using cold running water.
- Chop the cabbage head into blocks that will fit into the feeding chute of your juicer.
- Place the blocks of cabbage into your juicer then press down until fresh juice starts flowing.
- Keep adding blocks of cabbage until you have enough juice to fill one glass.

Apart from the weight-loss benefit of cabbage, this vegetable can also promote the health of your liver. When it comes to cleansing your liver, cabbage is considered a powerhouse as it contains vitamin C, sulfur, and potassium, all of which have detoxifying effects. Drink pure cabbage juice or add this vegetable in one of your juice blends to enjoy all the benefits!

Cucumber Juice

Fruits and vegetables that have high water content are typically low in calories—and cucumber is one such vegetable. By adding cucumber juice to your juicing regimen, you can promote weight loss. Just like the other juice options we have already discussed, this one can help you feel full for a longer time. Because of the high fiber and water content of cucumber juice, you will feel full after drinking one glass. To make it more palatable, you can add a squeeze of fresh lime or lemon juice and a couple of mint leaves to the fresh juice.

Cucumbers are one of the most common ingredients in salads because they are refreshing and they add a lovely crunch. But you can also enjoy cucumbers in juice form as part of your lineup of fresh juices. Here are the simple steps to follow for making cucumber juice with your juicer:

- Cut off the ends of the cucumber.
- You may or may not peel it before juicing. Either way, make sure to rinse the cucumber first before you start slicing.
- Cut the cucumber into pieces that will fit into the feeding chute of your juicer.
- Add pieces of cucumber into your juicer and press down until fresh juice starts flowing.
- If you don't mind the seeds, you can leave them in. Otherwise, you can use a cheesecloth to strain the seeds and only get pure juice.

Amazingly, one serving of cucumber juice contains less than 20 calories! And yet, you will already feel full after drinking the whole glass. You can make bigger batches of fresh cucumber juice to drink throughout the day. That way, you will only consume a few calories to help you reach your weight loss goals. This is particularly helpful when you embark on a juice cleanse.

Green Fruits and Veggies Juice Blend

This is a tasty detox juice blend that will fit in perfectly with your juicing regimen. It contains green apples and celery stalks that are high in fiber but low in calories, kale that has a low energy density, lemon that contains polyphenol antioxidants, ginger that has anti-inflammatory and antioxidant properties, and cucumbers, all of which work together to help you lose weight. The best part is, that this juice is super easy to make!

Nutritional Information: 150 kcal
Time: 6 minutes
Serving Size: 1 serving
Prep Time: 6 minutes
Cook Time: no cooking time
Ingredients:

- ½ lemon
- 1 cucumber
- 1 piece of ginger (fresh)
- 2 green apples
- 3 celery stalks (remove the leaves)
- a sprig of mint

Directions:

- Wash all of the fruits and veggies then use a paper towel to pat them dry.
- Peel the ginger, apples, cucumber, and lemon.
- Cut all of the ingredients into chunks that will fit into the feeding chute of your juicer.
- Place the fruit and vegetable pieces in your juicer. Press down on the juicer until fresh juice starts flowing. Juicing

the ingredients will depend on the type of juicer that you own.

- When you have enough juice to fill one glass, add the sprig of mint, and enjoy.

Roots, Leaves, and Fruits Juice Blend

Drinking this amazing juice blend is an excellent way for you to introduce fat-burning minerals, vitamins, and nutrients into your body. This detoxifying juice includes beets to help cleanse your liver and blood. This is an amazing benefit as a healthy liver metabolizes fats more effectively for faster weight-loss. It also contains oranges, which are high in fiber and vitamin C that promote fat-burning, especially in your belly, and pineapple that contains bromelain, a type of enzyme that promotes protein metabolism and fat-burning. Finally, this juice blend also contains high-fiber, low-calorie ingredients like cabbage, carrots, and lemon. It's chock-full of nutrients in a single glass.

Nutritional Information: approximately 357 kcal
Time: 6 minutes
Serving Size: 1 serving
Prep Time: 6 minutes
Cook Time: no cooking time
Ingredients:

- ¼ pineapple
- ½ lemon
- 1 medium beet
- 1 orange
- 2 red cabbage leaves
- 3 medium carrots
- a handful of spinach

Directions:

- Wash all of the fruits and veggies then use a paper towel to pat them dry.
- Peel the pineapple, lemon, beet, carrots, and orange.

- Cut all of the ingredients into chunks that will fit into the feeding chute of your juicer.
- Place the fruit and vegetable pieces in your juicer. Press down on the juicer until fresh juice starts flowing. Juicing the ingredients will depend on the type of juicer that you own.
- When you have enough juice to fill one glass, drink up!

Tropical Juice Blend

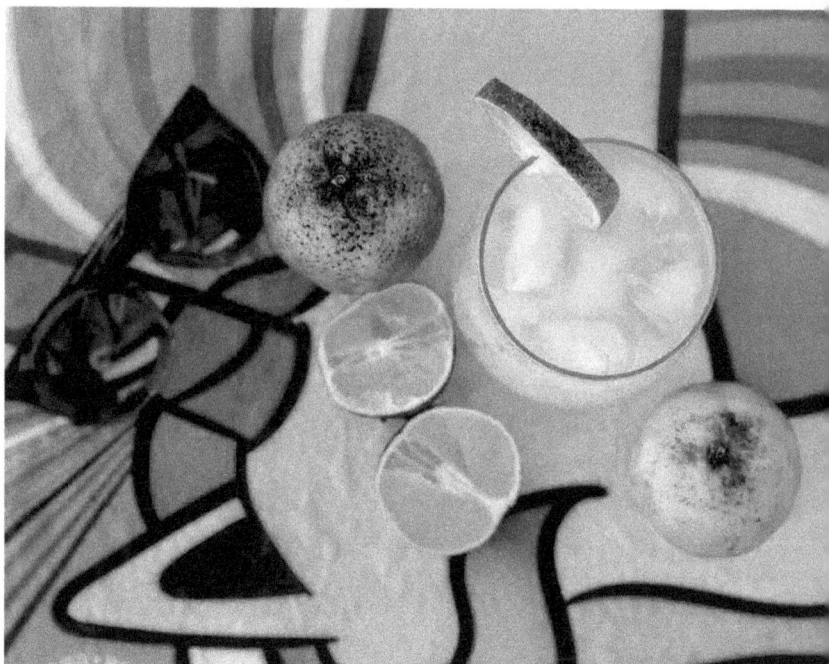

There's nothing more refreshing than a glass of fresh juice made from tropical fruits and veggies. Make your juice cleanse more interesting by including this recipe in your plan. It contains fresh apples, pineapples, carrots, and ginger, low-calorie ingredients that contain nutrients, vitamins, and minerals that will help you shed those stubborn excess pounds. The combination of this juice is amazingly perfect too!

Nutritional Information: approximately 224 kcal
Time: 5 minutes
Serving Size: 1 serving
Prep Time: 5 minutes
Cook Time: no cooking time

Ingredients:

- ½ cup of pineapple chunks
- 1 large apple
- 2 large carrots
- 2 pieces of ginger (fresh)

Directions:

- Wash all of the fruits and veggies then use a paper towel to pat them dry.
- Peel the apple, carrots, and ginger.
- Cut all of the ingredients (except the pineapple) into chunks that will fit into the feeding chute of your juicer.
- Place the fruit and vegetable pieces in your juicer. Press down on the juicer until fresh juice starts flowing. Juicing the ingredients will depend on the type of juicer that you own.
- When you have enough juice to fill one glass, you can enjoy your tropical juice blend.

Sweet and Tangy Juice Blend

Aside from helping you lose weight, this yummy juice blend will also calm your tummy. It contains a healthy combination of fruits and veggies to cleanse your digestive system and make it easier for you to shed excess pounds. As always, it's recommended to opt for organic produce, especially if you want to get all the benefits of juicing for weight-loss.

Nutritional Information: approximately 428 kcal
Time: 7 minutes
Serving Size: 1 serving
Prep Time: 7 minutes
Cook Time: no cooking time
Ingredients:

- 1 cup of spinach
- 1 cucumber
- 1 lime
- 1 piece of ginger (fresh)
- 2 celery stalks (remove the leaves)
- 3 medium apples

Directions:

- Wash all of the fruits and veggies then use a paper towel to pat them dry.
- Peel the cucumber, lime, ginger, and apples.
- Cut all of the ingredients into chunks that will fit into the feeding chute of your juicer.
- Place the fruit and vegetable pieces in your juicer. Press down on the juicer until fresh juice starts flowing. Juicing the ingredients will depend on the type of juicer that you own.

- When you have enough juice to fill one glass, enjoy this juice blend to calm your tummy, and make you feel better.

Orange Detox Juice Blend

Although orange in color, this isn't your ordinary glass of orange juice. It has a mild, sweet flavor that will surely make you feel satisfied. For this recipe, you will be using sweet potato that rehydrates the cells thanks to its high water content while boosting your body's metabolic activity. Although you can bake the sweet potato before juicing, you can also juice it raw just like all other fruits and veggies. Another unique ingredient you will find here is pear, which is rich in fiber while being low in calories—another weight-loss promoting fruit.

Nutritional Information: approximately 150 kcal
Time: 5 minutes
Serving Size: 2 servings
Prep Time: 5 minutes
Cook Time: no cooking time
Ingredients:

- 1 orange
- 1 sweet potato (around 5 inches long, either cooked or uncooked)
- 2 medium apples
- 2 medium pears
- 3 celery stalks (remove the leaves)

Directions:

- If you plan to cook the sweet potato, do this first.
- Wash all of the fruits and veggies then use a paper towel to pat them dry.
- Peel the orange, sweet potato, apples, and pears.
- Cut all of the ingredients into chunks that will fit into the feeding chute of your juicer.

- Place the fruit and vegetable pieces in your juicer. Press down on the juicer until fresh juice starts flowing. Juicing the ingredients will depend on the type of juicer that you own.
- When you have enough juice to fill one glass, enjoy this sweet, and filling juice blend.

Refreshing Juice Blend

Refreshing juice blends are the best because they make you feel full and... refreshed! Enjoy this healthy juice on a hot summer's day or on any other season of the year. Aside from the weight-loss benefit, this juice can help improve your complexion by promoting smooth, healthy skin. It will improve your skin's moisture while preventing blemishes. This means that it will refresh you from the inside-out.

Nutritional Information: approximately 877 kcal
Time: 7 minutes
Serving Size: 1 serving
Prep Time: 7 minutes
Cook Time: no cooking time
Ingredients:

- ½ cucumber
- ½ piece of ginger (fresh)
- 1 lemon
- 1 orange
- 3 celery stalks (remove the leaves)
- 3 medium apples
- 4 kale leaves

Directions:

- Wash all of the fruits and veggies then use a paper towel to pat them dry.
- Peel the cucumber, ginger, lemon, orange, and apples.
- Cut all of the ingredients into chunks that will fit into the feeding chute of your juicer.
- Place the fruit and vegetable pieces in your juicer. Press down on the juicer until fresh juice starts flowing. Juicing

the ingredients will depend on the type of juicer that you own.

- When you have enough juice to fill one glass, enjoy this refreshingly healthy juice blend.

Lemonade Blitz Juice Blend

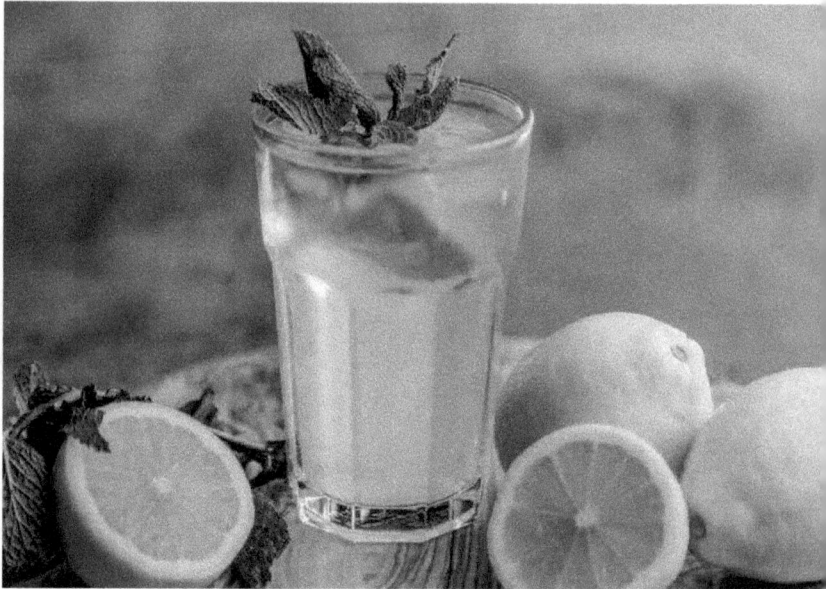

If you're looking for a tart, healthy juice blend, here's the best one for you. It contains a bunch of sour fruits along with some green veggies to make it healthier. If this juice blend is too sour for you, try adding a teaspoon of honey. You can also replace one of the green apples with a sweet, red apple to add sweetness to the mix. Either way, this juice is another winner when it comes to freshness and weight-loss benefits.

Nutritional Information: approximately 272 kcal
Time: 6 minutes
Serving Size: 1 serving
Prep Time: 6 minutes
Cook Time: no cooking time

Ingredients:

- 1 cup of spinach
- ½ lime
- 1 lemon
- 1 piece of ginger (fresh)
- 2 celery stalks (remove the leaves)
- 2 green apples
- 4 kale leaves

Directions:

- Wash all of the fruits and veggies then use a paper towel to pat them dry.
- Peel the lime, lemon, ginger, and apples.
- Cut all of the ingredients into chunks that will fit into the feeding chute of your juicer.
- Place the fruit and vegetable pieces in your juicer. Press down on the juicer until fresh juice starts flowing. Juicing the ingredients will depend on the type of juicer that you own.
- When you have enough juice to fill one glass, enjoy this tart, weight-loss promoting version of the classic lemonade drink.

Morning Glory Juice Blend

This juice blend is simple, sweet, and it's the perfect beverage to drink first thing in the morning. It's super easy to make and it's rich in the nutrients you need to lose weight. This cleansing juice blend will improve your liver's ability to fight fat while the high vitamin C content promotes fat-burning too, especially around your waist. By drinking this healthy juice blend, you can even improve your cholesterol. It even contains spirulina, a powerful superfood. What more should you ask for?

Nutritional Information: approximately 356 kcal
Time: 7 minutes
Serving Size: 1 serving
Prep Time: 7 minutes
Cook Time: no cooking time
Ingredients:

- 1 tsp spirulina (dried)
- 1 medium beetroot
- 2 medium carrots
- 2 oranges

Directions:

- Wash all of the fruits and veggies then use a paper towel to pat them dry.
- Peel the beetroot, carrots, and oranges.
- Cut all of the ingredients into chunks that will fit into the feeding chute of your juicer.
- Place the fruit and vegetable pieces in your juicer. Press down on the juicer until fresh juice starts flowing. Juicing the ingredients will depend on the type of juicer that you own.

- When you have enough juice to fill one glass, add the spirulina, mix well, and enjoy!

Red Hot Juice Blend

Are you ready for something healthy and spicy? This last recipe on our weight-loss juice list is not for the faint of heart. It contains the usual nutrient-dense ingredients plus one special ingredient to add a kick. For this recipe, you will be adding a jalapeño pepper that promotes fat-burning, boosts your metabolism, and reduces your appetite. It also gives this juice blend an interesting taste. If you want something to spice things up, add this to your juicing regimen too.

Nutritional Information: approximately 265 kcal
Time: 5 minutes
Serving Size: 1 serving
Prep Time: 5 minutes
Cook Time: no cooking time
Ingredients:

- 2 cups of spinach
- ½ lime
- 1 jalapeño
- 1 medium beetroot
- 1 piece of ginger (fresh)
- 2 celery stalks
- 5 large carrots

Directions:

- Wash all of the fruits and veggies then use a paper towel to pat them dry.
- Peel the lime, beetroot, ginger, and carrots.
- If you want to reduce the spiciness, you may de-seed the jalapeño first.

- Cut all of the ingredients (except the jalapeño) into chunks that will fit into the feeding chute of your juicer.
- Place the fruit and vegetable pieces in your juicer. Press down on the juicer until fresh juice starts flowing. Juicing the ingredients will depend on the type of juicer that you own.
- When you have enough juice to fill one glass, enjoy this unique juice blend with a kick.

Chapter 6:

Juicing Your Way to a Healthy Body

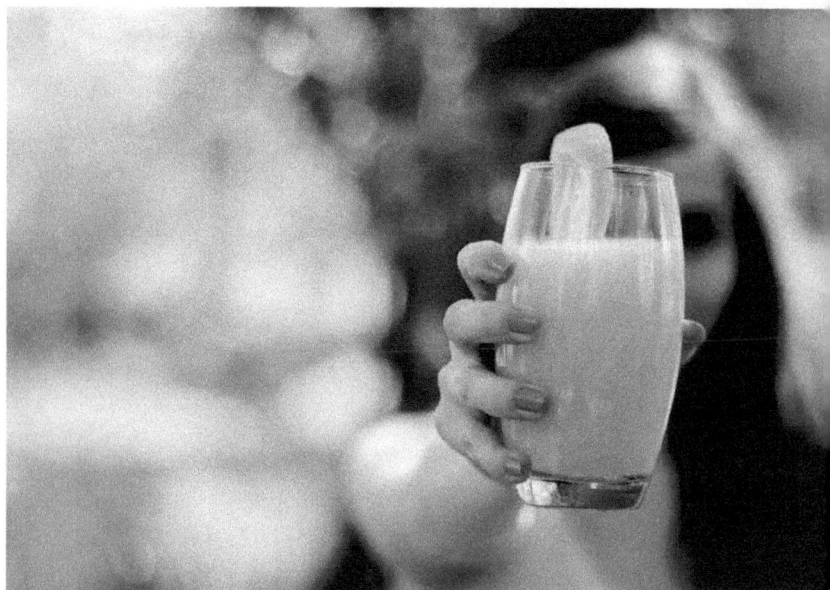

Fig. 14: Healthy Juice. Pixabay, by Jan Vašek, 2014,
https://pixabay.com/photos/orange-juice-healthy-glass-drink-569064/ Copyright 2014 by Jan Vašek/Pixabay.

Apart from weight loss, juicing offers a number of incredible health benefits, especially if you learn how to follow this detoxification process correctly. While a lot of people see juicing as nothing but a food trend, it does have a lot of promise. I have already shared my story with you and now, you are on your way towards embarking on your own juicing journey. In the last two chapters, you have learned all about how juicing promotes weight loss. Among all of the benefits of juicing, weight loss was the one that changed my life for the better.

When I started juicing, I might have been too focused on losing weight—so much that I didn't realize that this wasn't the only benefit juicing had to offer. In Chapter 1, I shared with you all of the wonderful benefits of juicing. Here, we will go review the most significant benefits, the ones that will truly help improve your overall health. But before moving forward, you should know that juicing isn't a 'quick-fix' to cure your illnesses and propel you to the peak of health. But it will put you on a path to achieving a healthier body if you do it correctly.

Now that you have a number of recipes that will help you lose weight, it's time to learn a couple of other recipes. The recipes here will help you target the health issues that you want to overcome or the aspects of your health that you want to focus on. After this, we can move on to helping you learn how to perform a proper juice cleanse, whether you are a juicing beginner or you have already tried juicing in the past.

The Health Benefits of Juicing

While a juice cleanse or a juice detox can help you lose weight, the health benefits go beyond this. In fact, if you try to focus on the wonderful changes that are happening to your body as you are juicing, you will realize that shedding a couple of pounds is just an added bonus that you will enjoy on top of the many health improvements you will experience. By doing regular juice cleanses, you will enjoy these health benefits long-term. As we have already discussed the most important health benefits in the second chapter, here are a few more to look forward to:

- Juicing will help transform your outlook on food. If you always had the tendency to choose unhealthy foods, regular juice cleanses will help you realize that choosing healthy foods makes you feel better—and this will encourage you to eat healthily.

- During your juice cleanse, your life becomes simpler as you won't have to think about the meals to cook or prepare for yourself. You would have already planned your juice cleanse so all you have to do is prepare your fresh juices.

- By drinking the right types of juice, you will notice your appetite getting smaller. Also, you will notice that you do not get cravings that lead you to binge eat, overeat or overindulge.

- Since the ingredients you will use to make fresh juices and juice blends are all healthy, your diet will get an amazing health boost. Because of this, you may notice that the health issues you have been experiencing will start fading away.

- Juicing improves the health of your liver. As you will help with the process of detoxifying your body, your liver gets a much-needed test. Since the liver is responsible for detoxification, drinking healthy juices and juice blends that fulfill the same purpose will make your liver healthier.

- Your body will thank you as you start juicing as you will experience a decrease in inflammation. Most vegetables have anti-inflammatory properties. Since most juice blends contain healthy veggies, you will get this benefit too.

With all of these health benefits to look forward to, it's no surprise that juicing will also improve your longevity. The healthier you are, the happier and longer you may live. Since juicing prevents diseases too, you won't have to worry about suffering through such ailments either.

To experience all of these benefits along with the ones featured in the previous chapters, you must first learn how to juice safely. Juicing isn't as simple as drinking a glass of juice once a day. You should always prioritize your health and to do this, you will learn the most effective juicing strategies in the next chapters. For now, let's go through the best types of juices and juice blend recipes to improve your health...

The Best Types of Juice for Blood Pressure Regulation

High blood pressure or 'hypertension' is becoming one of the most common health issues around the world and it often leads to a high mortality rate. By definition, hypertension is a condition wherein the force exerted by blood against the walls of your arteries is too high. The worst part is, both old and young people can develop this condition. If you don't do something about it, high blood pressure may lead to disastrous—even fatal—results.

Whether you are already suffering from hypertension or you feel like you have an increased risk of developing this condition, it's time for you to start making diet and lifestyle changes. You should avoid high-sodium foods, fatty foods, and fried foods. Instead, focus on following a diet that contains the right balance of protein, fiber, healthy fats, and complex carbs. Aside from this, you can start drinking different types of juices that can help regulate your blood pressure.

Beetroot Juice

Beetroot is an excellent source of nitrates that help relax your blood vessels to improve blood circulation. Although beetroot juice isn't the tastiest option out there, it works wonders in terms of blood pressure regulation. In fact, you can even feel this effect after drinking one glass of this juice a day. Beetroot also contains a wide range of nutrients and vitamins that promote the healthy function of blood. It also contains folate and potassium, both of which have a good effect on blood pressure. If pure beetroot juice doesn't agree with your taste buds, add some honey or any other type of natural sweetener to the mix. You can also add this ingredient to juice blends to mask its taste.

Cranberry Juice

Cranberries are considered a 'superfruit' because of their amazing antioxidant and anti-inflammatory properties. These properties will help prevent damage to your inner blood vessels to help lower your blood pressure. Cranberry juice can also dilate your blood vessels to make it easier for blood to flow through your body. This fruit also contains vitamin C, another nutrient that helps lower blood pressure naturally. The great thing about this juice is that you can drink it every day. Just stick with the fresh variety as most processed cranberry juices contain high amounts of sugar.

Pomegranate Juice

Here's another red-colored juice that will help lower your blood pressure naturally. Pomegranate juice can inhibit a specific enzyme known as angiotensin converting enzyme (ACE) that occurs in your body naturally. If you have high levels of this enzyme, you will experience elevated levels of blood pressure as it tends to tighten your blood vessels. Pomegranate juice works the same way as medications that doctors prescribe to lower blood pressure. This makes it a wonderful choice if you suffer from high blood pressure. As with beetroot juice, you can add natural sweeteners to the mix if you're making fresh pomegranate juice from home.

Spinach and Greens Juice

Spinach is one of the healthiest greens out there. Since it is rich in potassium, this veggie can help ease the tension in your arteries and blood vessels. This enhances the circulation of blood in your body to bring down your blood pressure to normal levels Spinach is also a great source of lutein which helps prevent the thickening of arterial walls to reduce the risk of high blood pressure. The other ingredients in this juice blend are excellent levels of potassium too making it one of the best options for you.

Nutritional Information: approximately 643 kcal
Time: 5 minutes
Serving Size: 1 serving
Prep Time: 5 minutes
Cook Time: no cooking time
Ingredients:

- 1 cup of spinach
- 1 piece of ginger (fresh)
- 2 stalks of celery (remove the leaves)
- 4 apples
- 4 lettuce leaves
- 6 carrots

Directions:

- Wash all of the fruits and veggies then use a paper towel to pat them dry.
- Peel the apples and carrots.
- Cut all of the ingredients into chunks that will fit into the feeding chute of your juicer.
- Place the fruit and vegetable pieces in your juicer. Press down on the juicer until fresh juice starts flowing. Juicing

the ingredients will depend on the type of juicer that you own.

- When you have enough juice to fill one glass, enjoy this juice blend that will help regulate your blood pressure levels.

The Best Types of Juice for the Immune System

Your immune system is one of the most important systems of your body as it protects you from diseases and infections. Because of this, you must do everything you can to promote the health of this essential bodily system. Fortunately, juicing can also strengthen your immune system as long as you pick the right ingredients for your fresh juices. Fruits and veggies contain immune-boosting vitamins that you can take advantage of. And since it's best to juice fruits and vegetables raw, you will surely get all the nutrients you need from them. While most fruits and veggies offer this benefit, here are some of the best options to include in your juicing regimen.

Citrus Juices

Citrus fruits are rich in vitamin C. This vitamin has antioxidant properties to protect your cells and bodily systems from harmful substances. By drinking fresh juice made from citrus fruits, you can prevent vitamin C deficiency. If you are deficient in this vitamin, your immune responses are impaired. This will lead to your body's inability to combat infections effectively. Instead of taking vitamin C supplements, drink fresh citrus juices to acquire this vitamin in the most natural and healthiest way possible.

Tomato Juice

Tomato juice is another excellent option, but not the processed kinds that are sold in stores. To get all of the immune-boosting benefits of tomato juice, you should make it yourself using fresh ingredients. It's super easy to juice tomatoes since they are already naturally juicy. So you would only need a couple of tomatoes to fill a glass. Tomatoes are an excellent source of folate that helps reduce your risk of developing infections. Tomatoes also contain magnesium that has anti-inflammatory properties.

ABC Juice Blend

A for apple, B for beet, and C for carrot. These three ingredients contain all of the nutrients that promote the health of your immune system. The combination of these ingredients makes for an interesting taste. It also includes ginger and lemon that add flavor and nutrition to the drink.

Nutritional Information: approximately 303 kcal
Time: 5 minutes
Serving Size: 1 serving
Prep Time: 5 minutes
Cook Time: no cooking time
Ingredients:

- 1 green apple
- 1 lemon
- 1 piece of ginger (fresh)
- 2 beets
- 3 carrots

Directions:

- Wash all of the fruits and veggies then use a paper towel to pat them dry.
- Peel the green apple, lemon, ginger, beets, and carrots.
- Cut all of the ingredients into chunks that will fit into the feeding chute of your juicer.
- Place the fruit and vegetable pieces in your juicer. Press down on the juicer until fresh juice starts flowing. Juicing the ingredients will depend on the type of juicer that you own.
- When you have enough juice to fill one glass, enjoy this healthy juice blend that promotes immunity.

Sunshine Juice Blend

This is a very simple juice blend that is healthy, fresh, and immunity-boosting. It contains only three ingredients but these ingredients are chock-full of nutrients that will help strengthen your body, especially your immune system. If you're in a rush but you want to have a fresh glass of juice, this is one of the best choices for you.

Nutritional Information: approximately 274 kcal
Time: 5 minutes
Serving Size: 1 serving
Prep Time: 5 minutes
Cook Time: no cooking time
Ingredients:

- 1 piece of ginger (fresh)
- 2 oranges
- 4 carrots

Directions:

- Wash all of the fruits and veggies then use a paper towel to pat them dry.
- Peel the ginger, oranges, and carrots.
- Cut all of the ingredients into chunks that will fit into the feeding chute of your juicer.
- Place the fruit and vegetable pieces in your juicer. Press down on the juicer until fresh juice starts flowing. Juicing the ingredients will depend on the type of juicer that you own.
- When you have enough juice to fill one glass, enjoy this fresh, sunny, immunity-boosting juice blend.

The Best Types of Juice for Better Digestion

Every time you start juice cleanses, your digestive system will thank you. Among all of the systems in your body, your digestive system is the one that will benefit the most because it will be able to rest and relax while you are juicing. Since there is no solid food to break down, most of your digestive processes will come to a halt—and this does wonders for your digestive health. As you drink juices and juice blends that contain digestive system-promoting ingredients, you will be boosting your digestive health even more.

Since fresh juices and juice blends contain high amounts of fiber, drinking these will help make you more regular in terms of your bowel movements. Rather than taking medications to overcome constipation, juicing is much healthier as it offers other benefits too. Juices also contain water, which means that they will contribute to your hydration throughout the day.

Lemon Juice

Fresh lemon juice is rich in vitamin C. This is an antioxidant compound that increases the amount of water in your gut to make your stool softer while stimulating the movement of bowels. Lemon juice is also refreshing, delicious, and hydrating which is why this is one of the most popular juice options around the world.

Prune Juice

Prune juice is quite famous for its laxative effects. By drinking prune juice regularly, you can help your digestive system improve its functions. You will notice improvements in terms of regular bowel movements, as well as, the consistency of your stool. Prunes contain high levels of dietary fibers along with potassium, magnesium, and sorbitol, all of which help give your bowel functions a boost.

Antioxidant Juice Blend

If you're looking for a juice blend that will calm your digestive system while flooding your body with antioxidants, this is the one for you. While this juice blend requires more preparation because it includes several ingredients, the benefits you reap from it will be well worth the effort. Aside from promoting better digestion, this juice blend will also boost the other systems of your body because of all the nutrients it contains.

Nutritional Information: 134 kcal
Time: 8 minutes
Serving Size: 1 serving
Prep Time: 8 minutes
Cook Time: no cooking time
Ingredients:

- 2 tsp apple cider vinegar (preferably organic with the 'Mother')
- ½ cup of parsley
- ½ beet
- 1 medium cucumber
- 1 small apple
- 1 small lemon
- 3 medium carrots
- 4 celery sticks
- ginger (fresh, you can add as much as you prefer)

Directions:

- Wash all of the fruits and veggies then use a paper towel to pat them dry.
- Peel the beet, cucumber, apple, lemon, and carrots.

- Cut all of the ingredients into chunks that will fit into the feeding chute of your juicer.
- Place the fruit and vegetable pieces in your juicer. Press down on the juicer until fresh juice starts flowing. Juicing the ingredients will depend on the type of juicer that you own.
- When you have enough juice to fill one glass, stir the apple cider vinegar in, and enjoy!

Go Green Juice Blend

If you suffer from any kind of digestive issue, this juice will help clear it up. It contains healthy ingredients that are rich in fiber to help regulate your bowel movements. Keeping this juice blend in your diet can even help reduce your risk of developing colon cancer. If you're a fan of fatty, spicy, and generally heavy foods, this is also an excellent option for you as it includes apples. This fruit contains enzymes that help your body digest fatty, spicy, and heavy foods. This juice blend also contains kale, which will help reduce the inflammatory effects of toxins on your digestive tract.

Nutritional Information: approximately 211 kcal
Time: 5 minutes
Serving Size: 1 serving
Prep Time: 5 minutes
Cook Time: no cooking time
Ingredients:

- 1 cucumber
- 1 green apple
- 1 lemon
- 5 kale leaves

Directions:

- Wash all of the fruits and veggies then use a paper towel to pat them dry.
- Peel the cucumber, apple, and lemon.
- Cut all of the ingredients into chunks that will fit into the feeding chute of your juicer.
- Place the fruit and vegetable pieces in your juicer. Press down on the juicer until fresh juice starts flowing. Juicing the ingredients will depend on the type of juicer that you own.

- When you have enough juice to fill one glass, enjoy this fresh juice blend that will improve your digestion.

The Best Types of Juice for Hormonal Regulation

Our hormones play a very important role in the different functions and processes in our body. This is why you will experience a number of health issues if even one of your hormonal levels is out of balance. Now, try to imagine what would happen if several of your hormones are thrown off balance. You will surely feel the adverse effects. Fortunately, one of the benefits of juicing is the regulation of hormones. Depending on the juice you drink or the ingredients you add to your juice blend, you can help your body get back on track by drinking fresh and tasty juice.

The great thing about juice is that it comes in liquid form, which is easy to absorb and digest by your body. This means that your hormonal health will improve quickly when you drink juices that contain vitamins, minerals, phytonutrients, and enzymes that support healthy cellular functions, especially in the hormonal cells and glands in your body.

Cruciferous Veggie Juice

This type of juice might seem strange but if you want to improve your hormonal health, you might want to make it part of your juice cleanse. Broccoli and other cruciferous veggies contain high levels of glucosinolates which have metabolism-altering properties when broken down. These will have an effect on specific hormones that cause diseases. You can make this juice more palatable by adding organic honey or even some kind of sweet fruit to the mix.

Sour Cherry Juice

Another unique choice, sour cherry juice contains high levels of melatonin and other phytochemicals that help improve your sleep. This is very important as getting enough high-quality sleep can help with hormonal regulation too. Since your body gets a chance to rest and repair itself while you are sleeping, getting enough sleep is crucial to improve your overall health too.

Herbed Fruit and Veggie Juice Blend

Herbs in your juice? Yes, please. This is another amazing juice blend that is both tasty and healthy, especially when it comes to hormonal regulation. In particular, the basil essential oil in this recipe can help balance your cortisol levels. Since cortisol is also known as the "stress hormone," it's important to bring balance to this hormone, especially when you're feeling stressed.

Nutritional Information: approximately 242 kcal
Time: 5 minutes
Serving Size: 1 serving
Prep Time: 5 minutes
Cook Time: no cooking time
Ingredients:

- ½ drop of basil essential oil
- 1 cup of kale leaves (chopped)
- 1 cup of pineapple (chopped)
- 1 lime
- 2 cucumbers
- 3 celery stalks

Directions:

- Wash all of the fruits and veggies then use a paper towel to pat them dry.
- Peel the lime and cucumber.
- Cut all of the ingredients into chunks that will fit into the feeding chute of your juicer.
- Place the fruit and vegetable pieces in your juicer. Press down on the juicer until fresh juice starts flowing. Juicing the ingredients will depend on the type of juicer that you own.

- When you have enough juice to fill one glass, add the basil essential oil to taste (and to add nutrition), and enjoy.

Orange-Colored Juice Blend

While this juice blend comes in a bright, orange color, it contains a wealth of ingredients that will help balance your hormones. It contains carrots that contain fiber, orange juice that contains vitamin C to help your adrenal glands produce hormones, beets that contain specific enzymes that aid in the elimination of toxins from your body (including excess hormones), and greens that improve all bodily processes including hormone functions.

Nutritional Information: approximately 370 kcal
Time: 10 minutes
Serving Size: 1 serving
Prep Time: 10 minutes
Cook Time: no cooking time
Ingredients:

- 2 cups of greens like kale and spinach (raw, organic)
- 1 beet
- 1 orange
- 1 small apple
- 3 carrots

Directions:

- Wash all of the fruits and veggies then use a paper towel to pat them dry.
- Peel the beet, orange, apple, and carrots.
- Cut all of the ingredients into chunks that will fit into the feeding chute of your juicer.
- Place the fruit and vegetable pieces in your juicer. Press down on the juicer until fresh juice starts flowing. Juicing the ingredients will depend on the type of juicer that you own.

- When you have enough juice to fill one glass, enjoy this juice blend right away for the best results.

The Best Types of Juice for Detoxification

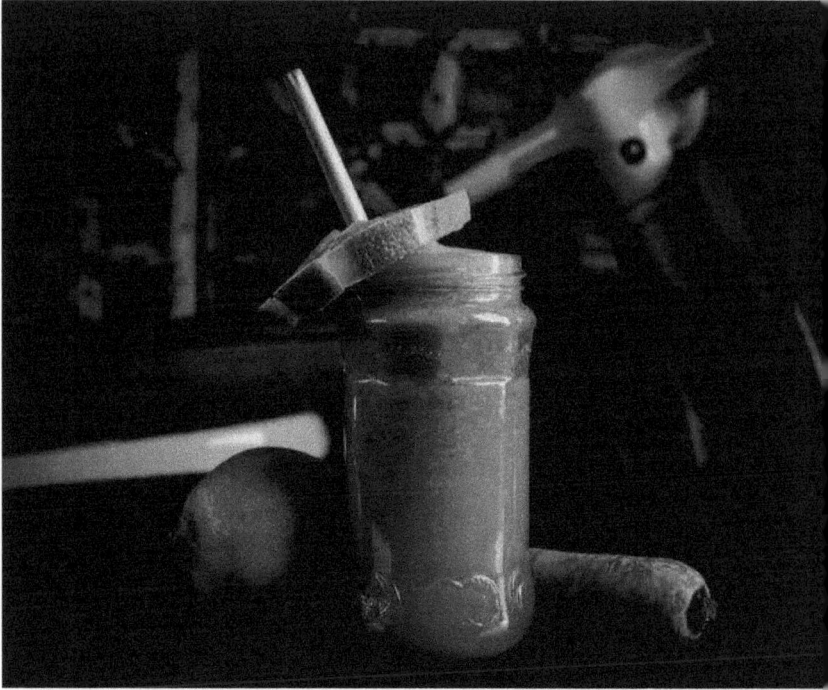

Fig. 15: Detox Juice. Unsplash, by Louis Hansel, 2018,
https://unsplash.com/photos/XG5JntFl2ws/ Copyright 2018 by Louis Hansel/Unsplash.

Detoxification is one of the most popular benefits of juicing. Although your body has a natural process of detoxification, you can improve this by drinking juice made from fresh fruits and vegetables. For this benefit, focus on produce that has anti-inflammatory and antioxidant effects as these are the ones that promote detoxification.

While helping to cleanse your body, these juices help your cells heal too. This is another amazing benefit as it improves the functions of cells. Imagine how healthy you will be when all of your cells are healthy and all of your bodily functions are running smoothly. Through juicing, you will feel rejuvenated and you can even avoid common diseases from developing.

Apple Juice

Apple juice is rich in vitamins, minerals, fiber, pectin, and phytochemicals, all of which promote the detoxification process. The acid content of apples helps with digestion while pectin helps flush out metals and additives from the body. If you really want to get all the benefits of apple juice, opt for organic apples for juicing.

Berry Juice

All types of berries like blueberries, blackcurrants, raspberries, and others are high in fiber and vitamin C. This means that drinking juice made from berries can help detoxify your body. The consumption of berries also stimulates your body to produce a fatty acid known as butyrate, which promotes weight loss by making your body leaner.

Detoxifier Juice Blend

As the name implies, this juice blend will detoxify your body and make it healthier. Whether you are performing a 3-day juice cleanse or you plan to stretch it to one week, don't forget to include this juice blend in your plan. This recipe makes a big batch of juice. After making it (and drinking one glass), you can store it in the refrigerator for an easy glass of juice without preparation.

Nutritional Information: approximately 121 kcal
Time: 10 minutes
Serving Size: 4 servings
Prep Time: 10 minutes
Cook Time: no cooking time
Ingredients:

- ½ lemon
- 1 piece of ginger (fresh)
- 2 medium apples
- 3 medium beets
- 6 carrots

Directions:

- Wash all of the fruits and veggies then use a paper towel to pat them dry.
- Peel the lemon, ginger, apples, beets, and carrots.
- Cut all of the ingredients into chunks that will fit into the feeding chute of your juicer.
- Place the fruit and vegetable pieces in your juicer. Press down on the juicer until fresh juice starts flowing. Juicing the ingredients will depend on the type of juicer that you own.

- When you have enough juice to fill one glass, enjoy this juice blend, and store the rest in your refrigerator for up to a week.

Ginger and Vegetable Zinger Juice Blend

This is another juice blend that will give you a zing but not as hot and spicy as the one you learned in the last chapter. The reason for this juice blend's 'zing' is the large quantity of ginger. Ginger is an important ingredient in detoxification as it is rich in antioxidants that will help reduce inflammation in your body. It contains other fresh ingredients that offer cleansing and detoxifying properties too.

Nutritional Information: approximately 175 kcal
Time: 8 minutes
Serving Size: 1 serving
Prep Time: 8 minutes
Cook Time: no cooking time
Ingredients:

- ½ cup of parsley
- 2 cups of spinach
- ½ cucumber
- ½ lemon
- 1 green apple
- 2 celery stalks
- 2 pieces of ginger (fresh)

Directions:

- Wash all of the fruits and veggies then use a paper towel to pat them dry.
- Peel the cucumber, lemon, apple, and ginger.
- Cut all of the ingredients into chunks that will fit into the feeding chute of your juicer.
- Place the fruit and vegetable pieces in your juicer. Press down on the juicer until fresh juice starts flowing. Juicing

the ingredients will depend on the type of juicer that you own.

- When you have enough juice to fill one glass and enjoy this juice blend chilled for the best results.

The Best Types of Juice to Help Slow Down the Aging Process

With all of the benefits you will experience through juicing, you will surely age gracefully. But wait, another benefit of juicing is to help slow down the aging process, which means that you won't have to worry about aging just yet if you start juicing regularly. The high antioxidant content of juices can help eliminate free radicals along with the most common signs of aging. These wonderful effects help prevent you from aging prematurely. As with the other health benefits, if you want to make the most of this one, pick your juices wisely.

Red Grape Juice

All parts of red grapes—even the seeds—have been used in beauty products to add an anti-aging property to them. This amazing benefit comes from the resveratrol content of red grapes. Resveratrol is an antioxidant that is very effective in combating the signs of aging. Make sure to include red grape juice in your juicing regimen whenever they are in season to help slow down your aging process.

Cucumber Juice

Cucumber is rich in a mineral called silicon which is vital for your body's connective tissues. By adding this mineral to your diet, you will also promote the health of your nails, hair, and skin. This means that cucumber juice is very beneficial in terms of anti-aging and an enhanced complexion. For the best results, drink a fresh glass of cucumber with ice.

Young and Fresh Juice Blend

Blueberries and apples are an amazing combination when it comes to ingredients that promote a youthful glow. These fruits are rich in pectin, antioxidants, and chlorogenic acids. This is a wonderfully tasty anti-aging juice blend that protects your brain and helps reduce aging lines from emerging on your skin. For a youthful glow and a sharp mind, prepare this juice blend now.

Nutritional Information: approximately 398 kcal
Time: 5 minutes
Serving Size: 1 serving
Prep Time: 5 minutes
Cook Time: no cooking time
Ingredients:

- 2 cups of apples
- 2 cups of blueberries

Directions:

- Wash all of the fruits then use a paper towel to pat them dry.
- Peel the apple and chop it into chunks that will fit into the feeding chute of your juicer.
- Place the fruits in your juicer. Press down on the juicer until fresh juice starts flowing. Juicing the ingredients will depend on the type of juicer that you own.
- When you have enough juice to fill one glass, enjoy this anti-aging juice blend.

Youthful Pink Juice Blend

Free radicals, stress, and not getting enough exercise or sleep can result in the development of wrinkles, age spots, and other signs of premature aging. The good news is that you can prevent these by adding more antioxidant-rich fruit and veggie juice blends to your diet. This is one such juice that includes healthy, youthful ingredients that produce a tasty, pink-colored juice blend when mixed together.

Nutritional Information: approximately 161 kcal
Time: 7 minutes
Serving Size: 1 serving
Prep Time: 7 minutes
Cook Time: no cooking time
Ingredients:

- ½ cup of strawberries
- 1 cup of blueberries
- 1 ½ cups of water (you may also use aloe vera juice)
- 1 large kale leaf
- 1 small beet

Directions:

- Wash all of the fruits and veggies then use a paper towel to pat them dry.
- Peel the beet and remove the stem of the kale leaf.
- Cut all of the ingredients into chunks that will fit into the feeding chute of your juicer.
- Place the fruit and vegetable pieces in your juicer. Press down on the juicer until fresh juice starts flowing. Juicing the ingredients will depend on the type of juicer that you own.

- When you have enough juice to fill one glass and enjoy this youthful juice blend that looks great and tastes even better.

Making the Most Out of Juicing for Your Health

Fresh fruits and vegetables are an essential part of a healthy, balanced diet. Sometimes, though, it can be very challenging to consume all of the fruits and veggies you need to stay healthy. The good news is that juicing can help you reach your diet goals. Juicing is an amazing supplement to a healthy diet. You can even perform regular juice cleanses to detoxify your body, lose weight, and enjoy other amazing benefits. If you want to make the most out of juicing for your health, here are some tips for you:

Learn How to Balance Your Nutrients

To enjoy all the benefits of juicing, learn how to incorporate it into a balanced diet. For one, you should try eliminating junk food from your diet before you start juicing, This is important, especially if you want to get rid of toxins in your body. Although juicing helps detoxify your body, consuming a lot of junk food, fast food, and processed food will counter the good effects of juicing. When this happens, it is unlikely that you will see good changes happening to your body—and you might not think that juicing is working.

You can also balance your nutrients by choosing your juicing ingredients carefully. For instance, if you only drink fruit juice, even if you make it from fresh fruits, your body will be getting high amounts of sugar and carbs. If your juicing regimen looks like this, you shouldn't expect to see beneficial results any time soon. Instead, learn how to make healthy juice blends and to create a schedule where you drink fresh fruit juices and vegetable juices too. This is particularly important if you are doing a juice cleanse. It's best to come up with a plan and a schedule first to ensure that your juice cleanse is nutritionally balanced.

Increase Your Vegetable Intake

One of the main benefits of juicing is to increase your veggie intake. You can make the most out of this by incorporating different types of vegetables in your juice blends. Pick the vegetables that you don't particularly like or those which you don't eat regularly. Combining these healthy vegetables with your favorite fruit will make it easier for you to consume. This is one of the best ways to add more veggies to your diet.

If you really want to boost your veggie intake, add a lot of green, leafy veggies to your juice blends. These are some of the healthiest veggies out there. They are low in carbs but high in fiber and other nutrients. Since most leafy vegetables are flavorless, adding them to your juice blends won't change the flavor but will give them a boost of nutrition.

Start Your Day With a Healthy Glass of Juice

Did you know that having a glass of juice for breakfast—or before breakfast—can flush out your digestive system? It will even give your body a powerful nutrient boost while giving you energy throughout the day. If you're always in a rush every morning, having a fresh glass of juice can be part of your routine. It's easy, convenient, and super healthy.

Have a Fresh Glass of Juice for Easy-to-Digest Nutrients

Although drinking juice in the morning is one of the healthiest ways you can have this beverage, you can also drink juice at any time of the day, especially if you need a quick boost of nutrition. For instance, if you're feeling tired or stressed, drink a glass of juice as a pick-me-up. Since juice is easily absorbed by the body, you will feel the effects right away. To get the most out of this, just make sure that you use the right ingredients for the type of juice blend you need.

Give Your Body Time To Process

Since juices and juice blends are rich in vitamins, minerals, and nutrients, it's best to drink on its own. This simply means that drinking a glass of fresh juice (especially a juice blend with several ingredients) might be too much for your body to process. When this happens, some of the nutrients might get wasted instead of being utilized by the body. To ensure that you're getting all of the healthy goodness, drink your glass of juice on an empty stomach. Then wait for about an hour before having a snack or meal to ensure that your body absorbs all of the nutrients from the juice first.

Drink Your Juice Right After Extracting It

Another way to get the most out of your drink is by drinking it right after you have extracted the liquid from fresh fruits and vegetables. This will give you the best flavor, the most appetizing appearance, and the highest nutritional value. The longer you let your glass of juice sit, the more enzymes get destroyed.

You Can Also Store Juice To Save Time

However, in some cases, you might not even have time to make fresh juice. Instead of buying processed juice from food shops, you can make bigger batches of juice then store the rest in your freezer. Pour the juice into freezer-quality storage bags then place these in your freezer. When it's time for you to drink, take a storage bag out of the freezer, and let the juice thaw naturally. While freezing destroys some of the enzymes, this option is still healthier than choosing store-bought products.

Opt for Organic Produce Whenever You Can

If you can find organic produce and if you can afford it, go for it! Organic produce doesn't contain chemical fertilizers and pesticides. This makes them significantly healthier. If you can't get a hold of organic fruits and veggies, visit your local farmers' market and choose regional, minimally-treated produce. Choose those which are in season as these tend to be cheaper too.

Add Some Protein To Your Juices

If you want to make your juice blends healthier, you can add some sort of protein to them. These may come in the form of supplements or specialized ingredients. Adding protein to your juices makes them healthier since fruits and veggies don't contain a lot of protein. Later, we will discuss the many options you can add to your juice blends.

Enjoy Both Juicing and Blending

Even though juicing is an amazingly beneficial process, you can also try blending fruits and veggies once in a while. Having a smoothie now and then will make you enjoy juicing more since smoothies are richer and have a different texture. Although juicing and blending are similar, the main difference between them is what you leave out. When you juice fruits and veggies, you are getting rid of all the fibrous materials so that you're only left with the liquid. But when you blend fresh fruits and veggies, you're using the fiber and pulp too. Either option is beneficial because:

- **Juicing**
  - Makes it very easy for your body to absorb nutrients.
  - Provides you with more concentrated amounts of nutrients, vitamins, and minerals.

- Lacks fiber, which makes it ideal for easier digestion, blood sugar regulation, and reducing the risk of developing heart disease.

- **Blending**
  - Includes more fiber, which helps improve digestion too.
  - Produces a denser beverage, which makes you feel fuller.

Once in a while, blend your fruits and veggies instead of juicing them. This makes things more interesting for you too.

Go Easy on the Fruits

When it comes to adding fruits to your juice blends to make them sweeter or more palatable, remember that a little goes a long way. Unless the recipe calls for different types of fruits or a large number of fruits (probably because of the nutrients they contain), you shouldn't add too many fruits to your juice blends. If you have whipped up a glass of juice and you don't like the taste, add juice from one fruit to the mix. Remember that you are juicing for your health, not to give yourself an excuse to drink sweet beverages.

Learn How To Pair the Right Ingredients

If you want to make delicious and healthy juice blends and extract all of the juice from your ingredients, juice firm, and flimsy ingredients together. For instance, if you're juicing green and leafy vegetables which are quite flimsy, pair these with firm ingredients like cucumbers, carrots or celery. This helps push all of the ingredients through your juicer, allowing you to extract all the juice you want.

When Drinking Dark-Colored Juice, Use a Straw

Healthy as juices are, some of them might end up staining your teeth. If you drink a lot of dark-colored juices and you drink these regularly, you might want to use a straw. That way, you can enjoy your tasty and healthy juice without compromising those pearly whites.

Think of Juicing as a Long-Term Thing

Unless you only plan to do juice cleanses once in a while, you may want to incorporate juicing into your daily routine to supplement your healthy, balanced diet. This will allow you to make the most out of juicing. In doing this, you will also increase your chances of enjoying the many benefits that juicing has to offer. The great thing about juicing is that it offers endless variety. You can even tweak some of the recipes you have learned here to make them taste better or make you feel fuller.

Whether you want to lose weight, cleanse your body, regulate your blood sugar levels or you're aiming for other health goals, juicing will help you out. Now that you know how to make the most out of juicing, you are well on your way to having the best juicing journey.

Chapter 7:

Preparing Yourself for the 7-Day

Juice Cleanse

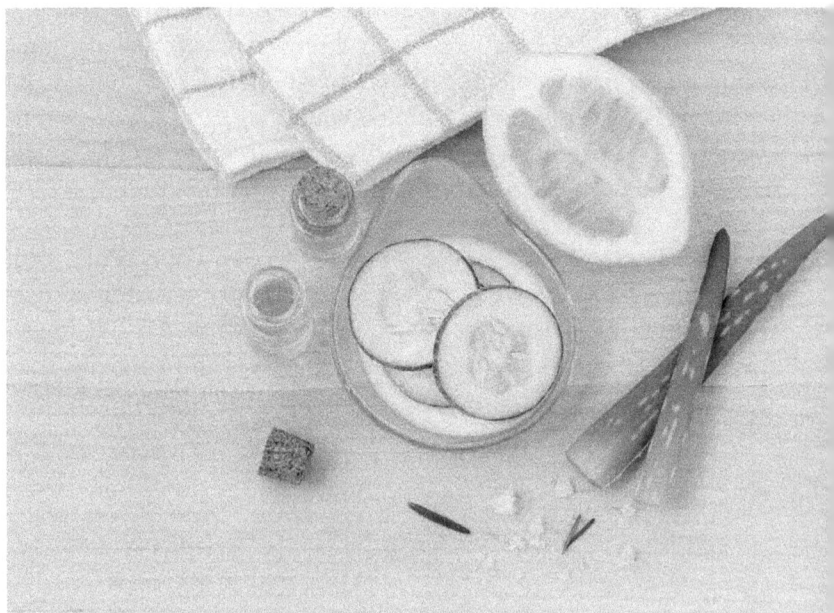

Fig. 16: Juice Cleanse. Pixabay, by Seksak Kerdkanno, 2015,
https://pixabay.com/photos/toner-skin-skincare-cooling-facial-906142/ Copyright 2015 by
Seksak Kerdkanno/Pixabay.

Have you ever wondered what it feels like to do a juice cleanse?
As someone who has performed plenty of juice cleanses already,
I can personally tell you that it feels amazing. These days, juice
cleanses have become quite popular. But if you want to make the

most out of them, you should know how to perform a juice cleanse correctly. A juice cleanse—also known as a juice fast or a juice detox—involves drinking fresh juices and juice blends that you have extracted from fresh ingredients. Throughout your juice cleanse, you will not be eating anything solid. Apart from juice, you can also drink other liquids like tea, water, and even clear broth.

If this is your first time to do a juice cleanse, you can start with a 3-day period. Since juice cleanses are quite intense because you won't be eating anything throughout the day, it's important for you to prepare for it. It's not something you decide on a whim as you might end up giving up on your juice cleanse on the first day. If you're interested in performing a juice cleanse, this is the most important chapter for you. Here, you will learn step-by-step instructions to help you plan, prepare, and perform your juice cleanse. No matter what your reason is for wanting to do regular juice cleanses, make sure that you are always doing them correctly. That way, you can ensure your safety and reduce the risk of experiencing potentially adverse side effects.

Who Should—and Should Not—Do a Juice Cleanse?

When it comes to juice cleanses, there really isn't a 'standard' way to do them. As long as you know what to avoid and how to approach this method safely, you can customize your plan to suit your own needs, preferences, and even your schedule. You can modify the recipes in the previous chapters to help you reach your health goals and create flavor combinations that cater to your personal preferences.

If you want to find success in juicing, you should enjoy it. Juicing shouldn't be something that you 'force' yourself to do, otherwise, it won't be sustainable for you. This is why you should try to be as flexible as possible without compromising your health. But before you start your very first juice cleanse, you should know that there are certain people who shouldn't be doing this mainly because of the potential health risks.

These people include:

- Children
- Pregnant women
- Breastfeeding women
- The elderly
- People with low blood sugar
- People with weakened immune systems
- People who suffer from diabetes
- People who suffer from chronic kidney problems
- People who are taking medications to treat chronic medical conditions

Also, if you suffer from any other type of medical condition or if you are currently taking medication, you must speak with your doctor first before planning your juice cleanse. If you're an adolescent or a parent with an adolescent who wants to try juice cleansing, it's recommended to speak with their doctor first. Just like young children, adolescents are still growing, and doing regular juice cleanses might inhibit their normal growth and development. The same thing goes if you are an athlete who participates in intensive training or sports activities. Athletes typically have very high-calorie needs because of the energy spent on training. By doing a juice cleanse while training or competing, you will not get all of the nutrients you need to recover properly.

Even if you are at the peak of your health, it's important to know that juice cleanses come with their own set of potential side effects. It's still important to be aware of these side effects in case you experience any of them during the course of your juice cleanse. That way, you won't start panicking then make an impulse decision to quit.

- **You may experience fatigue**

Since juices and juice blends contain lower amounts of fiber and higher amounts of sugar compared to whole foods, you may experience extreme fluctuations in your blood sugar levels, especially in the beginning. This might make you feel fatigued at some point. This is especially true for your first juice cleanse. Since your body isn't used to surviving on liquids alone, you might start feeling weak and tired. Of course, once your body gets used to the juice cleanse, then your blood sugar levels will stabilize and your energy levels will start rising too.

- **You may experience headaches**

Some experts believe that the headaches experienced by those who do juice cleanses are caused by the toxins that leave the body. However, the more likely causes are the low intake of energy and the fluctuations in blood sugar levels. As with fatigue, these headaches will soon fade when your body adjusts to the juice cleanse.

- **You may experience intense hunger**

This is the most obvious side effect since you will not be eating solids throughout the day. Again, this side effect is more likely to occur during your first few juice cleanses as your body learns to adjust to it. But if you perform juice cleanses regularly and you also drink fresh juice on the days when you aren't on a juice cleanse, you will soon get used to surviving on juice extracted from fresh ingredients.

Apart from these side effects, some people claim that one of the biggest downsides of juice cleanses is being very difficult to maintain. However, if you plan your juice cleanse well and you prepare yourself for it first, then you will surely find success. You should also approach juicing with a positive mindset so that you can keep yourself motivated throughout the process. Since this chapter is all about juice cleanses, you will learn what you need to keep yourself safe and healthy. And when you are done with your juice cleanse, make sure to follow a healthy, balanced diet to maintain a healthy and strong body.

Making the Most of Your Juice Cleanse

Lorem As you learn all about juice cleanses, you might feel like getting through three whole days of consuming nothing but juice seems like a scary, overwhelming goal. Yes, it is. And at some point, you might feel like giving up. Probably the best thing you can do when you do your first juice cleanse is to remind yourself of your goals. Remember why you have decided to do a juice cleanse in the first place. This will help keep you motivated even when things get tough.

When you go on a juice cleanse, you would only drink juice throughout the day for a set number of days. As a beginner, you should start with juice cleanses that only last between one to three days. After a couple of juice cleanses, you can increase the number of days gradually until you can handle a juice cleanse that lasts for seven days. To do a juice cleanse properly, you must go through the following stages:

- **Preparing for the Juice Cleanse**

  A few days before you start your juice cleanse, you should gradually eliminate foods and beverages like dairy products, meat, coffee, alcohol, wheat, and refined sugar. Doing this helps reduce your risk of experiencing withdrawal symptoms like cravings and headaches, for example. During the preparation stage, it would also be very helpful for you to increase your fluid, fruit, and vegetable intake.

- **Juice Cleanse**

  When you start your juice cleanse, you should have already prepared your plan for it. This includes how many days you plan to do your juice cleanse, what types of juices you will drink, and even a schedule to follow (although this can be flexible). During your juice cleanse, it's recommended that you drink a minimum of 32 ounces of smoothies or juice, half of which should consist of green, leafy veggies.

- **After the Juice Cleanse**

  After your juice cleanse, you shouldn't go back to your normal diet right away. A few days after the cleanse, you should gradually increase your food intake. This means that you start by eating lightly until you go back to your usual diet.

Simple, right?

The actual concept behind juice cleanses is very simple. But when it comes to making the most out of this detoxification process, there are many things you can do. Here are some tips for you:

- **Plan your meals during your preparation stage**

  Since the preparation stage occurs a few days before your actual juice cleanse, you should prepare for this too. Make sure to follow a light, balanced, and healthy diet at least three to five days before your juice cleanse. This will help ease your cravings and hunger pangs during your juice cleanse. When planning your meals, include a lot of fruits, veggies, and other healthy foods like eggs, whole grains, and a lot of water.

During this stage, you should also try to eliminate unhealthy foods like junk foods, fast foods, and processed foods from your diet. This will make it easier for your body to adjust to the juice cleanse. Basically, this stage serves as a 'pre-cleanse' wherein you are preparing your body for what will come next. If you can shift to a plant-based diet during this stage, even better! Just make sure to do this gradually.

By planning your meals, you won't have to make impulsive decisions, which may lead to indulging in heavy, unhealthy meals in the days leading up to your juice cleanse. Remember that this first stage is very important as it helps your body adjust to the juice cleanse. If you skip this step, you might experience adverse side effects like nausea, headaches, fatigue, and extreme hunger.

- **Prepare your recipes and ingredients**

After planning your meals for the preparation stage, it's time to plan your juice and juice blend recipes for the actual juice cleanse. Planning the recipes you will use makes it easier for you to reach your health goals. For instance, if you want to promote weight loss, there are certain types of juices and juice blends that can help you out. Include these in your plan to make it easier for you to cope during your juice cleanse.

When you have a plan for your juice recipes, it's time to choose the ingredients to use. As much as possible, opt for organic produce. Remember that organic fruits and veggies contain lower pesticide amounts. This is important since you will only be drinking juice made from these ingredients. If you want to be even more efficient, you can start preparing your ingredients too. You can purchase the ingredients, clean them, prepare them, and store them in the refrigerator properly. Then when it's time for you to make your juices, all you have to do is put the ingredients in your juicer and start the extraction process.

- **Make sure that you are still getting enough calories each day**

Since you will only be drinking fresh juice and other liquids during your juice cleanse, your body will already feel like it is being restricted. If you limit the amount of juice you drink in an attempt to hasten the weight loss process, this can be very dangerous to your health. Even if you are only drinking liquids throughout the day, make sure that you are still meeting your recommended caloric intake for the day. You can even add special ingredients and supplements to your juices to add protein. This ensures that your body gets the nutrition it needs even though you are only consuming juices, smoothies, and other liquids.

- **Keep yourself properly hydrated before, during, and after your juice cleanse**

While it is important to hydrate before and after your juice cleanse, this is even more important during the cleanse itself. You must drink more water during your juice cleanse so that you don't end up getting dehydrated. Drinking water can also eliminate your false hunger pangs by maintaining your cells' hydration.

When it comes to maintaining proper hydration, water is your best option. Try to avoid drinking highly caffeinated drinks like coffee or soda as these might mess with your body's alkalinity while you are on your juice cleanse. If you can't kick your coffee addiction, then you can opt for low-acid coffee. And try to keep your coffee intake to once each day during your juice cleanse.

- **Ease in—and out—of your juice cleanse**

  When you start your cleanse, it's important to ease into it. This is what the preparation stage is for. But when you are done with your juice cleanse, you should also ease out of it. This is where a lot of people make mistakes. After their juice cleanse, they immediately gorge on large meals of unhealthy foods. But when you do this, you might feel really bad afterward.

  As tempting as it is to binge on your favorite foods right after your juice cleanse, don't give in. You should give your body time to readjust by gradually introducing light meals to your diet. Just as you gradually eliminated certain foods from your diet as you prepared for your juice cleanse, you should also introduce those foods back into your diet gradually. Doing this will get your body used to digesting solids again to make it easier for you to go back to your normal diet.

- **Prepare yourself for the possible side effects**

  Juice cleanses may cause a number of side effects, especially during your first few times. Some of the more common side effects are fatigue, headaches, light-headedness, and even needing to sleep more. For the last one, you should listen to your body and try to get more sleep to optimize your juice cleanse. Since these are common side effects, then you might experience them too. Prepare yourself for them so that you don't get thrown off when they manifest. Learn how to listen to your body so that you don't overexert yourself or cause more harm to your body than good.

  Apart from the physical symptoms, prepare yourself for the emotional changes you may experience too. As you experience hunger pangs, lightheadedness, and all the other side effects of juice cleansing, these might make you feel unsure or even frustrated. Try to distract yourself by doing things that make you happy such as reading or watching movies, for example. These will make you feel better while reducing the stress you might feel because of your juice cleanse.

Another important tip to ensure that you make the most out of your juice cleanse is to slow down. Give yourself time to rest, observe your body, and reflect on the changes that you notice. If you are experiencing a stressful time in your life, don't start a juice cleanse as this might magnify your negative emotions. Instead, plan to have your juice cleanse on days when you know that you don't have a lot of things to deal with such as on weekends or vacations.

It would also be very helpful for you to start your juicing or juice cleanse journey with the right attitude. Before you start, you should already have your goals in mind. This gives you a purpose. When you have a purpose, you will feel more inspired and motivated to keep going no matter what challenges might come your way.

Safety Tips to Help You Thrive on the Juice Cleanse

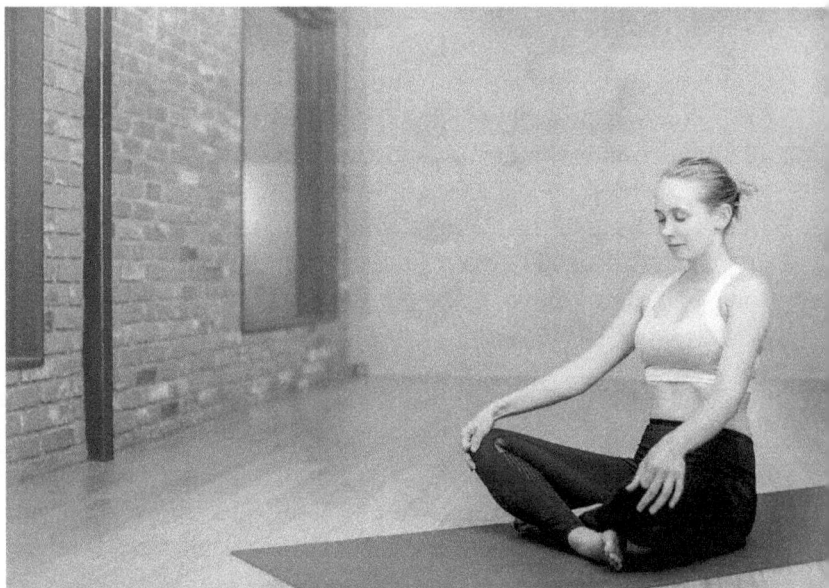

Whether you plan to start a new diet or you want to detoxify your body through a juice cleanse, your health and safety should always be your first priorities. Learning how to perform a juice cleanse correctly will help you get the results you are looking for without compromising your health. To help you survive your juice cleanse and thrive while doing it, here are some strategies for you:

Watch Your Workouts

Whether you're an athlete or a fitness enthusiast, you must tone down your workouts if you're planning to do a juice cleanse. Take a break throughout the duration of your juice cleanse. This doesn't mean that you shouldn't do any kind of exercise. If you really want to continue working out, stick with a light, low-intensity workout routine. This will be beneficial for you since exercising improves your respiration, blood circulation, and it makes you sweat. All of these will help the detoxification effects brought about by the juice cleanse.

During your juice cleanse, you can do light exercises like stretching or taking walks. While you are on a juice cleanse, expect your energy levels to change. Therefore, you should take your workouts down a notch (or a couple of notches if you're into high-intensity workouts) to avoid adverse side effects like lightheadedness or fatigue.

Pamper Yourself

Since you won't be working out as much, take this time to pamper yourself—and one of the best ways to do this is by taking a spa day. Whenever you perform a juice cleanse, you should also take some time off from your busy life. While your body is detoxifying from the inside, take some time to relax and do things that you have been putting off because you were "too busy" to do them. This is an amazing way to make your juice cleanse journey easier and more fun. By the end of your juice cleanse, you will feel refreshed, rejuvenated, and happier too.

Learn and Practice Mindfulness Techniques

Another thing you can do to make your juice cleanse easier and more effective is to find ways to nurture your mind too. While the juice cleanse promotes the wellness of your body, learning and practicing mindfulness techniques will promote the wellness of your mind. This is important since stress can have adverse effects on your health. Even if you're on a juice cleanse, if you are feeling stressed, this might impair the detoxification process. But if you combine your juice cleanse with meditation, gentle yoga routines, and other mindfulness techniques, you will surely experience all the wonderful benefits that juicing (and mindfulness) has to offer.

Encourage a Friend or Family Member to Join You

If you don't think that you can perform a juice cleanse on your own, encourage someone to join you. It can be a member of your family, a close friend or someone you can rely on to stick with you from start to finish. Having someone by your side who is taking the same journey as you can give both of you the motivation you need to keep going. Even if either of you experiences challenges, you can rely on each other to stay positive and make things easier for each other. If you can find a whole group of people to go on a juice cleanse with you, even better!

Don't Restrict Yourself Too Much

A juice cleanse is very simple—all you have to do is consume juice, smoothies, and other liquids throughout the day for a number of days. But if this is too much for you, especially if it is your first juice cleanse, don't force yourself to endure it. If you reach a point where you feel like you are going to faint if you don't eat something, allow yourself to have a light meal or snack.

In such a case, opt for organic veggies, fruits or even pre-soaked nuts. You can also drink meal replacement smoothies to overcome cravings and extreme hunger. Don't be too hard on yourself, especially during your first few juice cleanses. Otherwise, you might end up feeling too stressed or experiencing other adverse side effects. You want juicing to be a positive thing for you. And when you do give in, forgive yourself for it. Try not to feel guilty about eating something, especially if you ate something healthy and nutrient-dense.

Find Productive Ways to Distract Yourself

If you feel hungry during your juice cleanse (and you will!), try to find productive ways to distract yourself. Do something that makes you feel relaxed, catch up on your reading or even spend the whole day watching your favorite movies or TV series. However, you should try to avoid places with loud noises, lots of activities or even going out with friends to have a bite while you are doing your juice cleanse. It will be very stressful for you to sit in a restaurant while your friends eat scrumptious meals and all you have is a glass of juice. Again, it's all about trying to make your juice cleanse a positive experience. Do things that will help you associate juicing with happiness, relaxation, and fun.

Drink as Much as You Need

Remember the tip about getting enough calories throughout the day? Before you start your juice cleanse, you must first determine the optimal quantity of juice you should drink each day—and make sure to stick with that amount. If you feel like you are still hungry, opt for healthy liquids like water and broth.

Don't Rush Into Things

If this is your first time to do a juice cleanse, try it out for a day or two, three days at most. Doing this will give you a better idea of how it feels. It will also give you an idea of whether you can increase the number of days already or not yet. As time goes by, you can continue increasing the number of days until you are strong enough to do a 7-day juice cleanse. When you do decide to do a juice cleanse, don't forget the preparation stage as this helps your body adjust to the detoxifying process to increase your chance of completing your juice cleanse without a hitch.

Learn How to Listen to Your Body

If you want to get the most out of juicing and juice cleanses while staying safe, you must learn how to listen to your body. Even if you follow all of the suggested tips, you should observe your body while you are juicing. This is the best way for you to determine if you are experiencing any adverse side effects. In such a case, you may decide whether you will continue with the juice cleanse to see if you will feel better, make adjustments to your strategies or ease out of the juice cleanse, and come up with a new plan. Listening to your body is the most effective way to stay safe so this is something that you must learn.

Get Enough Sleep

Since a juice cleanse involves only consuming liquids for a number of days, you need to get enough sleep to help your body recover. When I say sleep, you shouldn't just aim for enough hours. You should also make sure that you are getting quality sleep each night. If you don't have one yet, come up with a bedtime routine to help you relax and fall asleep easily at night. Try to sleep at the same time each night and get up at the same time each morning. And about one hour before turning in, put your phone away. Spend time doing relaxing activities so that you will stay asleep throughout the night from the moment you fall asleep.

When it comes to juicing and juice cleanses, accept that things will not always be perfect. There might be times that you will experience challenges even if you think you have planned everything perfectly. Be kind to yourself and practice flexibility. This will help you succeed as you will start seeing this healthy process as something that will improve your health. After internalizing all of these safety tips and strategies, here is one last thing for you to do...

Know the Risks and Try to Avoid Them

Juicing isn't a one-size-fits-all solution to your health problems nor is it a diet that will help you achieve your health goals right away. Juicing is a process that takes time, effort, and the right strategies to get right. Just like any other changes you make in your diet, juicing comes with its own risks. By being aware of these risks, you can try to avoid them while performing your juice cleanses:

- **Decreased nutrition**

  Although fresh juices and juice blends are rich in nutrients, you will still be eliminating solid foods from your diet during juice cleanses. This will definitely decrease your nutrition. This is why you shouldn't perform a juice cleanse for too many days. While juicing can supplement your healthy diet, juice cleanses aren't something you should do long-term. When you're done with your juice cleanse, gradually ease back into your healthy, balanced diet then drink fresh juice regularly to increase your fruit and veggie intake.

- **Lack of healthy fats and fiber**

  Most fruits and veggies are naturally low-fat. While this might sound like a good thing, your diet should also include healthy fats as these play an important role in nerve function, nutrient absorption, skin, hair, and nail health, hormone production, and disease prevention. As you go back to your normal diet, make sure to include healthy fat sources too.

  Although fresh fruit and vegetable juices contain fiber, you aren't getting all of the fiber content from the fresh ingredients because most of the fiber comes from the seeds, skin, and pulp. To get more fiber into your diet, you should also try to increase your consumption of whole fruits and veggies, especially when you're not doing juice cleanses.

- **Lean muscle loss**

    Another nutrient that fruits and proteins aren't that rich in is protein. This macronutrient is important for the repair, support, and maintenance of your muscles. If you only drink juice and nothing else for long periods of time, your body won't have enough protein to keep functioning well. When this happens, it might start consuming protein from your muscles, which will then lead to lean muscle loss. As with fiber, healthy fats, and other nutrients, make sure to get enough protein from lean and healthy protein sources.

As you can see, it isn't that difficult to avoid the potential health risks that come with juicing. The key is to stick with a healthy, balanced diet so that juicing will support and complement your diet to improve your overall health.

A Sample 3-Day Juice Cleanse for Beginners

As a juicing beginner, you should be very careful with how you plan and execute your very first juice cleanse. Ideally, you would start juicing to supplement your diet to help you get used to preparing and drinking fresh juice. When it's time for you to do a 3-day juice cleanse, you won't be eating anything throughout those days. It might sound overwhelming and even while you are doing it, you might get overwhelmed. But if you can stick with it for three whole days, then you would have successfully helped your body eliminate the toxins that have accumulated from the food you eat.

Before you start preparing the ingredients for your juices and juice blends, you may want to create a schedule for the whole duration of your juice cleanse. In Chapter 5 and Chapter 6, you have been introduced to several juices and juice blend recipes that offer different benefits. You may start by including those suggestions in your plan. Since you already have recipes, the next thing to prepare is your schedule. For each of the three days, your schedule can look like this:

- **7:00 am to 8:00 am (right after you wake up):** Start your day with a warm or lukewarm glass of water with fresh lemon juice.
- **9:00 am to 10:00 am:** Have a glass of pure vegetable or fruit juice OR a juice blend that includes fresh fruit and vegetable juices.
- **10:30 am to 11:30 am:** Have a glass of pure vegetable or fruit juice OR a juice blend that includes fresh fruit and vegetable juices OR a smoothie for something heavier/more filling.
- **1:00 pm to 2:00 pm:** Have a glass of pure vegetable or fruit juice OR a juice blend that includes fresh fruit and vegetable juices OR a smoothie for something heavier/more filling.
- **3:00 pm to 4:00 pm:** Have a glass of pure vegetable or fruit juice OR a juice blend that includes fresh fruit and vegetable juices.
- **5:00 pm to 6:00 pm:** Have a glass of pure vegetable or fruit juice OR a juice blend that includes fresh fruit and vegetable juices OR a smoothie for something heavier/more filling.
- **7:00 pm to 9:00 pm:** Have a juice blend that includes fresh fruit and vegetable juices OR a smoothie for something heavier/more filling OR a glass of nut milk.
- **10:00 pm to 11:00 pm (right before going to bed):** End your day with a warm or lukewarm glass of water with fresh lemon juice.

If you want to optimize your body's absorption of the nutrients in the juices, you should drink each glass slowly instead of gulping everything down. As you can see with the schedule above, you will be drinking juices, smoothies, and even milk throughout the day. In between these schedules, if you feel hungry, you can drink a glass of water or consume a bowl of broth if you're craving something savory.

During your first few juice cleanses, you may want to print out your schedule including the juice recipes that you plan to drink throughout the day. This will make it easier for you to do the juice cleanse properly for the entire duration. The great thing about juice cleanses is that you can make adjustments to your schedule or plans as needed. If you discover that something isn't working, change it! And if you discover some juices or juice blends that you really find appealing and palatable, take note of these. Include them in your next juice cleanses so that you always have something to look forward to.

A 3-day juice cleanse is perfect for beginners as it allows you to detoxify your body without feeling like you're pushing yourself too hard. During the juice cleanse, you may experience hunger, cravings, and headaches. As long as these aren't too intense, try to stick with your juice cleanse until you complete the three days. Then you can gradually reintroduce solid foods into your diet until you finally go back to your normal eating habits. Only this time, you should continue your juicing journey as a supplement to your diet.

A Sample 7-Day Detox Juice Cleanse for Those with Experience

After you have performed 3-day juice cleanses for a few times, you can gradually increase the number of days. For instance, after doing 3-day cleanses three times, the next time you do a juice cleanse, increase the number of days to four. Keep doing this until you feel like you are ready to perform a 7-day juice cleanse. As someone who has been doing 7-day juice cleanses regularly for some time now, here is a schedule and plan that works for me—and that might work for you too:

Day 1

- **6:00 am to 7:00 am (right after you wake up):** Start your day with a warm or lukewarm glass of water with fresh lemon juice.
- **8:00 am to 9:00 am:** Have a glass of pure vegetable juice for breakfast. Some of the best options are beetroot, carrots, celery, coriander, kale, mint, parsley, spinach or wheatgrass. If you want to add a boost of fiber to your veggie juice, add one tablespoon of chia seeds, and mix well before drinking.
- **10:00 am to 11:00 am:** Have a glass of pure vegetable or fruit juice OR a juice blend that includes fresh fruit and vegetable juices OR a smoothie for something heavier/more filling.
- **12:30 pm to 1:30 pm:** Have a glass of pure vegetable or fruit juice OR a juice blend that includes fresh fruit and vegetable juices OR a smoothie for something heavier/more filling.
- **2:30 pm to 3:30 pm:** Have a glass of pure vegetable or fruit juice OR a juice blend that includes fresh fruit and vegetable juices.
- **4:30 pm to 5:30 pm:** Have a glass of pure vegetable or fruit juice OR a juice blend that includes fresh fruit and vegetable juices OR a smoothie for something heavier/more filling.
- **7:00 pm to 9:00 pm:** Have a juice blend that includes fresh fruit and vegetable juices OR a smoothie for something heavier/more filling OR a glass of nut milk.
- **10:00 pm to 11:00 pm (right before going to bed):** End your day with a warm or lukewarm glass of water with fresh lemon juice OR a cup of unsweetened herbal tea.

If you feel like you need to eat something, you may have lightly steamed veggies like beetroot, broccoli, cabbage, carrots, fenugreek leaves, mushrooms, mustard leaves, pumpkin or spinach. Throughout the day, don't forget to drink water. You may also have unsweetened herbal tea if you prefer.

Day 2

- **6:00 am to 7:00 am (right after you wake up):** Start your day with a warm or lukewarm glass of water with fresh lemon juice.
- **8:00 am to 9:00 am:** Have a glass of pure vegetable juice for breakfast. Some of the best options are beetroot, carrots, celery, coriander, kale, mint, parsley, spinach or wheatgrass. If you want to add a boost of fiber to your veggie juice, add one tablespoon of chia seeds, and mix well before drinking.
- **10:00 am to 11:00 am:** Have a glass of pure vegetable or fruit juice OR a juice blend that includes fresh fruit and vegetable juices OR a smoothie for something heavier/more filling.
- **12:30 pm to 1:30 pm:** Have a glass of pure vegetable or fruit juice OR a juice blend that includes fresh fruit and vegetable juices OR a smoothie for something heavier/more filling.
- **2:30 pm to 3:30 pm:** Have a glass of pure vegetable or fruit juice OR a juice blend that includes fresh fruit and vegetable juices.
- **4:30 pm to 5:30 pm:** Have a glass of pure vegetable or fruit juice OR a juice blend that includes fresh fruit and vegetable juices OR a smoothie for something heavier/more filling.

- **7:00 pm to 9:00 pm:** Have a juice blend that includes fresh fruit and vegetable juices OR a smoothie for something heavier/more filling OR a glass of nut milk.
- **10:00 pm to 11:00 pm (right before going to bed):** End your day with a warm or lukewarm glass of water with fresh lemon juice OR a cup of unsweetened herbal tea.

If you feel like you need to eat something, you may have lightly cooked veggies with quinoa. A salad that contains baby spinach would also be a great snack. Throughout the day, don't forget to drink water. You may also have unsweetened herbal tea if you prefer.

Day 3

- **6:00 am to 7:00 am (right after you wake up):** Start your day with a warm or lukewarm glass of water with fresh lemon juice OR a cup of unsweetened herbal tea.
- **8:00 am to 9:00 am:** Have a glass of pure vegetable juice for breakfast. Some of the best options are beetroot, carrots, celery, coriander, kale, mint, parsley, spinach or wheatgrass. If you want to add a boost of fiber to your veggie juice, add one tablespoon of chia seeds, and mix well before drinking.
- **10:00 am to 11:00 am:** Have a glass of pure vegetable or fruit juice OR a juice blend that includes fresh fruit and vegetable juices OR a smoothie for something heavier/more filling.
- **12:30 pm to 1:30 pm:** Have a glass of pure vegetable or fruit juice OR a juice blend that includes fresh fruit and vegetable juices OR a smoothie for something heavier/more filling.
- **2:30 pm to 3:30 pm:** Have a glass of pure vegetable or fruit juice OR a juice blend that includes fresh fruit and vegetable juices.
- **4:30 pm to 5:30 pm:** Have a glass of pure vegetable or fruit juice OR a juice blend that includes fresh fruit and vegetable juices OR a smoothie for something heavier/more filling.
- **7:00 pm to 9:00 pm:** Have a juice blend that includes fresh fruit and vegetable juices OR a smoothie for something heavier/more filling OR a glass of nut milk.
- **10:00 pm to 11:00 pm (right before going to bed):** End your day with a warm or lukewarm glass of water with fresh lemon juice.

If you feel like you need to eat something, you may have half a cup of plain Greek yogurt with chia seeds and walnuts or sliced almonds. You may also have a light salad made with organic ingredients if you're craving something savory. Throughout the day, don't forget to drink water. You may also have unsweetened herbal tea if you prefer.

Day 4

- **6:00 am to 7:00 am (right after you wake up):** Start your day with a warm or lukewarm glass of water with fresh lemon juice OR a cup of unsweetened herbal tea.
- **8:00 am to 9:00 am:** Have a glass of pure vegetable juice for breakfast. Some of the best options are beetroot, carrots, celery, coriander, kale, mint, parsley, spinach or wheatgrass. If you want to add a boost of fiber to your veggie juice, add one tablespoon of chia seeds, and mix well before drinking.
- **10:00 am to 11:00 am:** Have a glass of pure vegetable or fruit juice OR a juice blend that includes fresh fruit and vegetable juices OR a smoothie for something heavier/more filling.
- **12:30 pm to 1:30 pm:** Have a glass of pure vegetable or fruit juice OR a juice blend that includes fresh fruit and vegetable juices OR a smoothie for something heavier/more filling.
- **2:30 pm to 3:30 pm:** Have a glass of pure vegetable or fruit juice OR a juice blend that includes fresh fruit and vegetable juices.
- **4:30 pm to 5:30 pm:** Have a glass of pure vegetable or fruit juice OR a juice blend that includes fresh fruit and vegetable juices OR a smoothie for something heavier/more filling.

- **7:00 pm to 9:00 pm:** Have a juice blend that includes fresh fruit and vegetable juices OR a smoothie for something heavier/more filling OR a glass of nut milk.
- **10:00 pm to 11:00 pm (right before going to bed):** End your day with a warm or lukewarm glass of water with fresh lemon juice.

If you feel like you need to eat something, you may have an extra smoothie that contains bananas, yogurt, and chia seeds. You may also have a bowl of organic vegetable stew. Throughout the day, don't forget to drink water. You may also have unsweetened herbal tea if you prefer.

Day 5

- **6:00 am to 7:00 am (right after you wake up):** Start your day with a warm or lukewarm glass of water with fresh lemon juice.
- **8:00 am to 9:00 am:** Have a glass of pure vegetable juice for breakfast. Some of the best options are beetroot, carrots, celery, coriander, kale, mint, parsley, spinach or wheatgrass. If you want to add a boost of fiber to your veggie juice, add one tablespoon of chia seeds, and mix well before drinking.
- **10:00 am to 11:00 am:** Have a glass of pure vegetable or fruit juice OR a juice blend that includes fresh fruit and vegetable juices OR a smoothie for something heavier/more filling.
- **12:30 pm to 1:30 pm:** Have a glass of pure vegetable or fruit juice OR a juice blend that includes fresh fruit and vegetable juices OR a smoothie for something heavier/more filling.

- **2:30 pm to 3:30 pm:** Have a glass of pure vegetable or fruit juice OR a juice blend that includes fresh fruit and vegetable juices.
- **4:30 pm to 5:30 pm:** Have a glass of pure vegetable or fruit juice OR a juice blend that includes fresh fruit and vegetable juices OR a smoothie for something heavier/more filling.
- **7:00 pm to 9:00 pm:** Have a juice blend that includes fresh fruit and vegetable juices OR a smoothie for something heavier/more filling OR a glass of nut milk.
- **10:00 pm to 11:00 pm (right before going to bed):** End your day with a warm or lukewarm glass of water with fresh lemon juice OR a cup of unsweetened herbal tea.

If you feel like you need to eat something, you may have half a light salad. Although by the fifth day, you should have already overcome your cravings or hunger pangs. Throughout the day, don't forget to drink water. You may also have unsweetened herbal tea if you prefer.

Day 6

- **6:00 am to 7:00 am (right after you wake up):** Start your day with a warm or lukewarm glass of water with fresh lemon juice.
- **8:00 am to 9:00 am:** Have a glass of pure vegetable juice for breakfast. Some of the best options are beetroot, carrots, celery, coriander, kale, mint, parsley, spinach or wheatgrass. If you want to add a boost of fiber to your veggie juice, add one tablespoon of chia seeds, and mix well before drinking.
- **10:00 am to 11:00 am:** Have a glass of pure vegetable or fruit juice OR a juice blend that includes fresh fruit and vegetable juices OR a smoothie for something heavier/more filling.
- **12:30 pm to 1:30 pm:** Have a glass of pure vegetable or fruit juice OR a juice blend that includes fresh fruit and vegetable juices OR a smoothie for something heavier/more filling.
- **2:30 pm to 3:30 pm:** Have a glass of pure vegetable or fruit juice OR a juice blend that includes fresh fruit and vegetable juices.
- **4:30 pm to 5:30 pm:** Have a glass of pure vegetable or fruit juice OR a juice blend that includes fresh fruit and vegetable juices OR a smoothie for something heavier/more filling.
- **7:00 pm to 9:00 pm:** Have a juice blend that includes fresh fruit and vegetable juices OR a smoothie for something heavier/more filling OR a glass of nut milk.
- **10:00 pm to 11:00 pm (right before going to bed):** End your day with a warm or lukewarm glass of water with fresh lemon juice OR a cup of unsweetened herbal tea.

If you feel like you need to eat something, you may have a bowl of vegetable soup or a bowl of broth. Throughout the day, don't forget to drink water. You may also have unsweetened herbal tea if you prefer.

Day 7

- **6:00 am to 7:00 am (right after you wake up):** Start your day with a warm or lukewarm glass of water with fresh lemon juice OR a cup of unsweetened herbal tea.
- **8:00 am to 9:00 am:** Have a glass of pure vegetable juice for breakfast. Some of the best options are beetroot, carrots, celery, coriander, kale, mint, parsley, spinach or wheatgrass. If you want to add a boost of fiber to your veggie juice, add one tablespoon of chia seeds, and mix well before drinking.
- **10:00 am to 11:00 am:** Have a glass of pure vegetable or fruit juice OR a juice blend that includes fresh fruit and vegetable juices OR a smoothie for something heavier/more filling.
- **12:30 pm to 1:30 pm:** Have a glass of pure vegetable or fruit juice OR a juice blend that includes fresh fruit and vegetable juices OR a smoothie for something heavier/more filling.
- **2:30 pm to 3:30 pm:** Have a glass of pure vegetable or fruit juice OR a juice blend that includes fresh fruit and vegetable juices.
- **4:30 pm to 5:30 pm:** Have a glass of pure vegetable or fruit juice OR a juice blend that includes fresh fruit and vegetable juices OR a smoothie for something heavier/more filling.
- **7:00 pm to 9:00 pm:** Have a juice blend that includes fresh fruit and vegetable juices OR a smoothie for something heavier/more filling OR a glass of nut milk.
- **10:00 pm to 11:00 pm (right before going to bed):** End your day with a warm or lukewarm glass of water with fresh lemon juice.

If you feel like you need to eat something, you may have some grilled organic veggies or a bowl of broth. Throughout the day, don't forget to drink water. You may also have unsweetened herbal tea if you prefer.

After the seventh day, you're done! Now all you have to do is gradually reintroduce solid foods into your system. Remember to do this gradually so that you don't end up feeling bloated or sick afterward. When it comes to 7-day cleanses, here are some tips for you along with some things to keep in mind:

- While this schedule includes some healthy snack options, it's better to do a complete juice cleanse. You should only opt for the snack suggestions if you feel like you cannot go through with the whole process. Instead of giving up, allow yourself to eat something healthy.
- When choosing the juices and juice blends to incorporate into your 7-day schedule, choose wisely. Make sure that the recipes you choose will help you reach your health goals. Also, try to find the right balance of juices to drink throughout the day. For instance, it isn't recommended to only drink pure fruit juices throughout the day as this might mess up your blood sugar levels.
- As you try different juice recipes, adjust them according to your own tastes and preferences. As long as you don't add too many fruits to your juices, you can tweak the recipes a bit to make them more palatable for you.
- By the time you do a 7-day juice cleanse, this means that you would have already done several juice cleanses. This means that you can start experimenting with recipes. Find out which ingredients will help you lose weight or reach other health goals then use those ingredients to create interesting combinations.

If you have successfully completed your 7-day juice cleanse without giving in to your hunger or cravings, good for you! Now it's time to start going back to your normal diet. Since you have skipped solids for a whole week, be very careful with how you break your juice cleanse. You may want to start with small, light salads, and fresh fruits before you move up to cooked foods that contain protein, healthy fats, and other non-plant-based foods. Also, this would be the perfect time to start cleaning up your diet so that your health will continue to improve over time.

Chapter 8:

Making Lifestyle Changes to

Complement Your Juice Cleanse

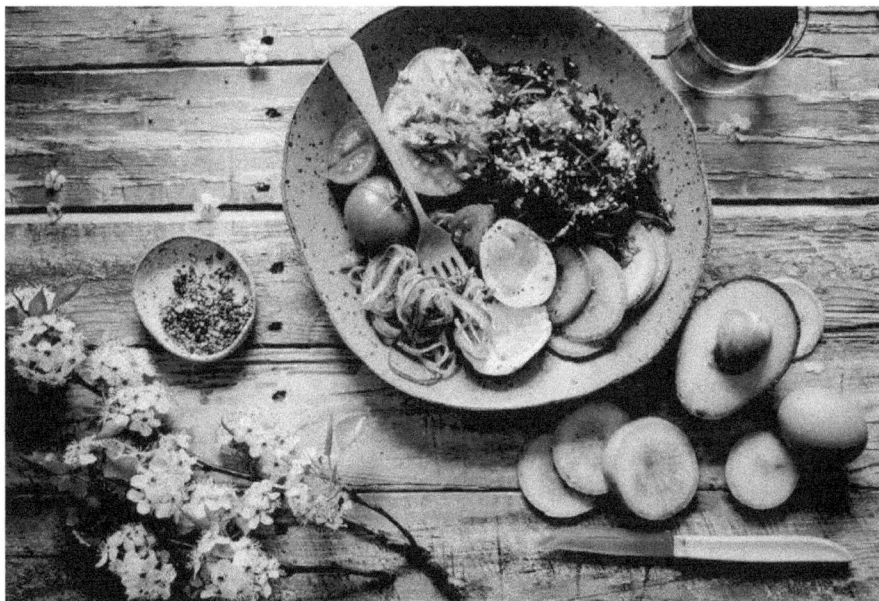

Fig. 18: Healthy Diet. Unsplash, by Brooke Lark, 2017,
https://unsplash.com/photos/jUPOXXRNdcA/ Copyright 2017 by Brooke Lark/Unsplash.

If you want juicing to become a beneficial part of your life, you should complement it with positive changes to your lifestyle. These include a healthier diet, regular exercise, and even breaking unhealthy habits like smoking or excessive alcohol consumption. In this final chapter, we will go through all of the lifestyle changes you should make to improve your health and enhance the effects of juicing.

Healthy Ingredients and Superfoods to Add to Your Juice Blends

When whipping up juices and juice blends, you can add a number of superfoods to make them healthier, tastier, and more filling. The ingredients that you add to your juice depends on the flavor you want, the benefits you're looking for, and the ingredients that you have already added to your juice. Here are some of the best and healthiest superfoods you may consider:

- **Apple Cider Vinegar**

  Apple cider vinegar has a lovely sour taste to complement different types of juice blends. It offers probiotic and anti-inflammatory properties to improve your health. It can also help balance your pH levels to provide relief from the symptoms of acid reflux. Just make sure to look for organic apple cider vinegar with the 'Mother.' This ingredient is best added to juice blends that contain apples, cucumbers, and pears.

- **Aloe Vera**

  Aloe vera is a succulent plant that has a high phytochemical content that helps improve your immune system while cleansing your blood. It also offers anti-inflammatory properties while improving your body's ability to absorb nutrients. This ingredient is best added to juice blends that contain honeydew, cucumbers, and pears.

- **Bee Pollen**

  Bee pollen offers a lot of health benefits including weight loss. It also helps decrease gastrointestinal problems, improves athletic performance, and relieves the symptoms of PMS. Just make sure that you aren't allergic to bee pollen before adding it to your juices. Bee pollen has a sweet taste making it a great combination with different juice blends, especially when combined with cinnamon.

- **Cayenne**

  Cayenne is a hot spice that contains capsaicin, a powerful anti-inflammatory compound. It also contains nutrients that help boost your immune system. Since this ingredient is quite spicy, don't add too much right away. It's best to add small amounts of cayenne to your juice, so you don't ruin the whole drink. If you think that you want more spice, then you can add more as needed. Because of its taste, you can add this ingredient to veggie-based juice blends.

- **Chia Seeds**

  Chia seeds are an excellent source of fiber and omega-3 fatty acids. They even have the potential to lower your blood pressure and cholesterol levels. If you add chia seeds to your juice, remember that they tend to swell after a couple of minutes. If you don't like this texture, drink your juice right away. Chia seeds add some nuttiness to your juice blends so they go well with any types of juices or smoothies.

- **Chlorella**

  Chlorella is a potent superfood that offers a number of health benefits. This is a nutrient-dense freshwater alga that usually comes in the form of a tablet or a powder. It's high in fiber, protein, antioxidants, and healthy fats, which is why it has become a very popular food supplement. Add a spoonful of this ingredient to your juice or smoothie for a healthy nutrient boost.

- **Cinnamon**

  Cinnamon is a great addition to any juice as it tastes great and it helps manage your cholesterol and blood sugar levels. This spice contains an antioxidant known as cinnamic acid that helps prevent the oxidation of omega-3 fatty acids. If you're making smoothies, you can add a cinnamon stick to your blender. But if you're making juice blends, ground or freshly grated cinnamon are better options.

- **Coconut Oil**

  Coconut oil helps improve thyroid function while balancing your blood sugar levels. It also offers antioxidant, anti-viral, and anti-fungal properties. It's best to add melted coconut oil to your juices as you might not appreciate its texture when chilled. Coconut oil adds a mild flavor and it goes well with juices that contain tropical fruits.

- **Flax Seeds**

  Flax seeds are rich in omega-3 fatty acids and fiber to improve your cardiac health. These tiny seeds also contain lignans to help prevent your risk of cancer. Although you may add flax seeds to your juices, it's better to add ground seeds as these are easier for your body to absorb. This ingredient has a slightly grassy and nutty flavor making it suitable for different types of juice blends.

- **Hemp Seeds**

  Hemp seeds are becoming more popular these days as a health supplement even though they are quite controversial. Although hemp seeds come from the marijuana plant, they don't contain high levels of THC—the compound that makes you high. Instead, hemp seeds contain omega-6 and omega-3 fatty acids that help lower blood pressure and cholesterol levels. These nutty seeds contain a lot of fiber and protein too. Adding them to your drinks will give you a huge nutrient boost. Whether you are preparing juices or smoothies, hemp seeds are an amazing addition.

- **Maca Powder**

  Maca powder is made from a Peruvian root that also comes in the form of a fermented drink. It helps improve mood, energy, and even fertility. Dried maca powder stores well and has a very long shelf life. With its nutty flavor, you can add maca powder to your juices to increase your endurance, energy, and bring balance to your hormone levels. To enhance the benefits, combine maca powder with flax seeds in your juice drinks.

- **Nutritional Yeast**

  Nutritional yeast is also called brewer's yeast. This amazing superfood is rich in B vitamins, minerals, and protein. You can add it to your juices either in powder form or as flakes. Although very healthy, this ingredient has a bitter taste so you shouldn't add too much to your juice. Adding nutritional yeast gives a unique flavor that's somewhat savory so it's best added to juices like orange, apple, carrots or spinach.

- **Protein Powder**

Protein powder is one of the most common ingredients added to juices and smoothies, especially for those who are focused on their health. There are many types of protein powders to choose from, either plant-based or animal-based. By adding this ingredient to your juice, it helps repair and rebuild muscles, making it ideal if you work out regularly.

- **Raw Cacao Nibs**

Raw cacao nibs will add a chocolatey taste to your juices with a hint of bitterness. These nibs contain monounsaturated fats, minerals, flavonoids, and antioxidants. They also contain protein making them an amazing supplement to add a boost of nutrition to your juice blends. You can either purchase whole nibs to grind at home or you can buy raw cacao nibs in powder form to add directly to your drinks.

- **Spirulina**

Spirulina is a type of algae that can help heal different types of illnesses from liver disorders to allergies, and even oral cancer. This ingredient is rich in minerals, antioxidants, vitamins, and amino acid proteins. It's best added to green juices and smoothies to make them even healthier. At first, you might not appreciate the taste of spirulina, but you don't have to add a lot of the powdered form to get all the health benefits it has to offer. Although spirulina is best added to green juices and smoothies, you can also add it to other types of juices like carrot, beet, and apple, for example. Keep using spirulina in different juice blends to get used to the flavor or to find the best combinations that mask the taste of this healthy superfood.

- **Turmeric**

Turmeric is a root from India that has a similar appearance as ginger. It contains potent antioxidant properties along with other amazing nutrients. Turmeric helps promote the healthy metabolism of carbohydrates and fats while offering anti-inflammatory properties too. Turmeric has a piquant flavor making it perfect for green smoothies and juices or drinks that contain pineapple or carrots.

- **Walnuts**

Walnuts are high in protein just like all other nuts. This ingredient superfood is rich in omega-3 fatty acids and monounsaturated fats too. Walnuts also contain a B-complex vitamin known as biotin that contributes to the health of your skin, nails, and hair while strengthening your body's ability to process fatty acids. You can add whole walnuts when processing smoothies in a blender after soaking them in water first. Grind walnuts and add to your juices for a grainy texture and a nutrient boost. This ingredient is great with juices and smoothies that contain blueberries, bananas, and other fruits.

- **Wheatgrass**

Wheatgrass is another superfood that offers immune-system boosting and anti-inflammatory properties. This ingredient also contains vitamin A, vitamin B, vitamin C, vitamin E, and a host of healthy minerals. You can drink wheatgrass juice on its own or add it to smoothies for a healthier drink. As with some of the other superfoods on our list, this one has a taste that you have to get used to. But when you consider all of the nutrients it contains, you'll know why adding this ingredient to your juices is a must. The best types of juices you can add wheatgrass to are those which contain banana and pineapple. You can even add some type of nut milk or coconut water to the mix for a refreshing and healthy beverage.

As you can see, there are so many different types of ingredients and superfoods you can add to your juices to make them healthier and more interesting. As with fruits and veggies, experiment with these different ingredients to see which ones you like and which ones will help you reach your health goals faster.

Diet Tips to Help You Out

Juice cleanses can feel overwhelming but if you can get through them, you will surely feel healthier and more rejuvenated after. In itself, juicing is already very healthy. But if you pair juicing with a healthy and balanced diet, you can improve your health in countless ways. To ensure your success on your juicing journey, here are some diet tips to guide you:

- **Opt for whole foods**

  This means that you should opt for foods that don't contain preservatives and added sugar. It's best to eat these before and after your juice cleanse but even if you aren't planning a juice cleanse, you should still focus on whole foods like fruits and veggies. Even though processed foods are tastier and more convenient, whole foods will help you achieve your health goals and maintain your health after reaching those goals. As you follow your normal diet, aim to consume at least three to five servings of veggies and two to three servings of fruit each day. Then you can supplement your diet with fresh juices to increase your nutrient intake and improve your health.

- **Make sure you're getting healthy fats**

When people hear the word 'fat,' they immediately think of gaining weight. Because of this, most people try to eliminate fats from their diets completely. However, your body needs healthy fats to survive and thrive. Some of the best sources of healthy fats include olive oil, avocadoes, nuts, and other plant-based foods. You can also get healthy fats from fatty fish like salmon and sardines. Aside from providing you with health benefits, healthy fats also make you feel fuller and more satisfied so you don't end up overeating at every meal or eating snacks too frequently.

- **Probiotics can improve your health too**

Consider introducing more probiotic-rich foods to your diet, especially if you believe that your gut flora is out of balance. Greek yogurt, fermented veggies or cultured veggies are some of the best sources of probiotics. These foods are easy to digest and they offer amazing benefits to your digestive system. It's particularly beneficial for you to consume probiotic-rich foods right after your juice cleanse.

- **Stay away from sugar, caffeine, and alcohol**

Before, during, and after your juice cleanse, you should eliminate sugar, caffeine, and alcohol from your diet. In particular, your body finds it difficult to digest refined sugars so you should stay away from these as much as possible. If you're craving something sweet, opt for fruits instead.

You should also avoid caffeinated beverages, especially before and during your juice cleanse. After your juice cleanse, gradually reintroduce caffeinated beverages into your diet so you don't end up messing with your sleeping schedule. Alcoholic beverages are also discouraged, especially in excessive amounts. Before and during your juice cleanse, you shouldn't drink alcohol. After your juice cleanse, you should wait for a few days before reintroducing alcohol into your system.

- **Always stay hydrated**

  Whether you are planning a juice cleanse, doing a juice cleanse or you are following your normal diet, staying hydrated is essential. This helps improve your digestive processes while keeping all of your other bodily systems running smoothly too.

- **Eat small meals regularly throughout the day**

  If you plan to incorporate juicing into your diet, it's recommended to eat small meals throughout the day instead of eating heavy meals at different times throughout the day. If you can drink a glass of juice before your meals, this will make it easier for you to lose weight as you will be eating smaller portions too.

When doing a juice cleanse, it's important to plan how you will reintroduce foods into your diet after your juice cleanse. Transitioning back to your normal diet shouldn't be done impulsively. Remember—you would have eaten nothing during your juice cleanse, only liquids. If you eat a huge meal on the first day after your juice cleanse, there is a very high likelihood that you will end up experiencing adverse side effects afterward. On the first day right after your juice cleanse, your meals might look like this:

- Your first breakfast can either be a light bowl of fruits or a light salad that consists of dark, leafy green veggies. This meal will help maintain the balance of your pH levels that you achieved through your juice cleanse.
- Your first lunch can be more substantial but still not heavy. You can have a smoothie along with a light meal like steamed fish with a side of veggies. As soon as you feel full, stop eating.
- Your first dinner is when you can have some carbs to boost your energy. Opt for healthy carbs like black beans, brown rice or quinoa combined with fresh veggies and olive oil.

After the first day, you can systematically reintroduce other foods like meat and dairy to your diet. As you do this, observe how your body reacts to the new foods. If you notice any adverse side effects, take note of these. You can also start eating different types of nuts as healthy and filling snacks. After your first day, the next few days of your post-cleanse might look like this:

- **On the second day**
    - Continue consuming small portions of quinoa or other types of healthy carbs.
    - Continue eating whole fruits, veggies, and healthy fat sources like avocados, peanut butter, and nuts.
    - Start introducing starchy veggies into your diet.
    - Maintain proper hydration throughout the day.

- **On the third day**

- Continue eating fruits, veggies, healthy fats, and healthy carbs.
- Start introducing dairy products into your diet slowly.
- Start introducing easy-to-digest animal proteins like eggs, lean chicken, and tofu.
- Maintain proper hydration throughout the day.
- Start drinking small amounts of caffeinated beverages if desired.

- **On the fourth day and beyond**
  - Continue eating fruits, veggies, healthy fats, and healthy carbs.
  - Maintain proper hydration throughout the day.
  - Continue introducing more types of foods to your diet, but not too many varieties each day.

Juicing and juice cleanses work best when paired with healthy diets. Even if you aren't following a healthy, balanced diet right now, you can start juicing while you are transitioning into this type of diet. Just make sure that you have fully transitioned into a healthier diet before you plan to do your first juice cleanse.

Exercises on a Juice Cleanse

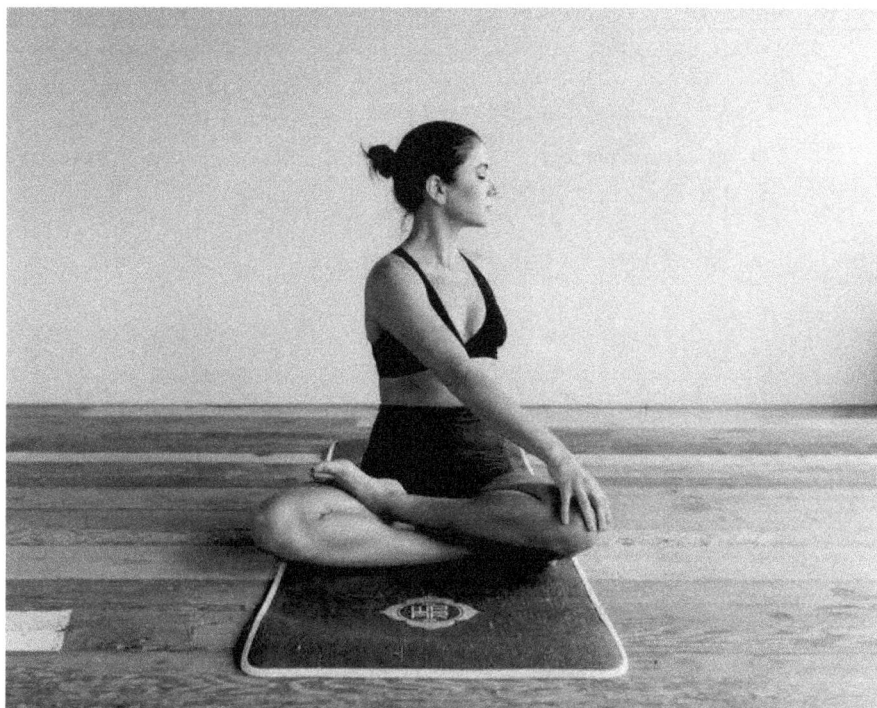

Fig. 19: Exercises. Unsplash, by Dane Wetton, 2019,
https://unsplash.com/photos/t1NEMSm1rgI/ Copyright 2019 by Dane Wetton/Unsplash.

Just because you are on a juice cleanse, doesn't mean that you have to stop exercising. If you're doing a 1-day juice cleanse, then you may choose to take a day off from your workouts. But if you're planning to do longer juice cleanses and you don't want to give up your workout regimen, all you have to do is take things down a notch. This is especially true if you want to nourish and detoxify your body while allowing yourself to repair and heal. In such a case, you should focus more on rest and relaxation instead of trying to maintain your intense workouts.

The best type of workouts to do during your juice cleanses are low-impact exercises. These will help relax your body and mind while still allowing you to maintain physical activity. Also, low-impact exercises will help improve the detoxification process. For instance, stretching and deep breathing exercises help eliminate toxins from your body. When you pair these exercises with your juice cleanse, you will surely see better results. Apart from stretching and deep breathing, here are other exercises for you to try:

- **Light Cycling or Jogging**

  If you are into intense workouts, these are probably the most intense types of workouts you can do while on a juice cleanse. But if you plan to go cycling or jogging, you may want to increase the protein content of your juices. You can add supplementary superfoods to your juices and smoothies like chia seeds or protein powder, for example. This will help your body keep up with the workouts you are doing while on the juice cleanse.

- **Walking**

  Walking is a natural activity that we all do. But when you increase your pace, this helps oxygen pump through your blood and lungs more efficiently to enhance your body's detoxifying abilities. Walking is a relaxing activity too, so it's perfect for when you're on juice cleanses.

- **Yoga**

  Yoga is another amazing low-impact workout that you can do while on juice cleanses. Yoga allows you to stretch your muscles, relax your mind, improve your balance, and increase your breathing capacity. This relaxing activity can be a permanent part of your healthy lifestyle along with a healthy diet supplemented with juicing.

While the mere idea of taking your workout routines down a notch might seem troublesome for you, just think of it this way: you will only do your juice cleanse for a few days. You don't have to give up exercising. You just have to slow down, relax, and allow your body to rejuvenate through the healthy juices that you consume.

In fact, for the first few days of your juice cleanses—or during your first few juice cleanses—you might not even have the strength to do your high-intensity workouts. Even if you consume juices and smoothies that you supplemented with protein-rich superfoods, these still won't be enough to sustain intense physical activity. If you try to force yourself to do these workouts, then you might end up feeling dizzy or fatigued. Then you might feel discouraged from doing juice cleanses in the future. Give yourself a break and allow yourself to slow down... your body will thank you for it.

Whether you choose to continue with low-impact workouts or you choose to give yourself a complete break, make sure that you are drinking enough juice throughout the day. Even without physical activity, your body still needs nutrients to survive. Even if weight loss is your main goal, you should still drink sufficient amounts of juice throughout the day. You might think that drinking less juice will help you lose more weight but you might end up compromising your body if you do this. Since you won't be eating anything during your juice cleanse, you will definitely lose weight. You don't have to take things further by reducing your juice intake too. This might even push you to overeat once your juice cleanse ends.

If regular exercise isn't part of your daily routine, you should consider starting now. Exercise is an essential part of a healthy life. You can start by doing simple exercises like stretching, walking, and yoga. As time goes by, you can increase the intensity of your exercises to improve your body's fitness. And each time you plan to do a juice cleanse, adjust your workout routines accordingly.

Making the Right Lifestyle Changes

Apart from exercising regularly and following a healthy diet, there are certain lifestyle changes you can make to improve the effects of juicing. Remember that juicing isn't something that you do for a few weeks or months then give up. It's something that you can incorporate into your daily routine to make sure that your body is always getting enough fruits, veggies, and nutrients each day. There are so many lifestyle changes you can make and here are some of the best ones:

Try Infrared Saunas to Promote Further Detoxification

Have you ever tried going into a sauna? If you have, you would know how relaxing saunas can be. However, infrared saunas differ from traditional saunas as they won't heat the air that surrounds you. Infrared saunas involve the use of infrared lamps that emit electromagnetic radiation to directly warm your body up. This makes it easy to penetrate the tissues in your body so that your body heats up faster than the air around you. Detoxification is one of the main benefits of infrared saunas but they can also provide relief from pain and soreness, better sleep, tighter and clearer skin, relaxation, improved circulation, and even weight loss. Once in a while give this type of sauna a try to improve your health and make you feel rejuvenated.

Consider Skin Brushing to Strengthen Your Lymphatic System

Skin brushing or dry brushing is a health practice that is typically offered in spas. This process involves brushing your skin using a dry brush while following a specific pattern. After the skin brushing process, you would then take a shower. For this process, you would start from your hands and feet going towards your chest, and heart. Skin brushing is an amazing process that offers a number of benefits such as lymphatic strengthening and support, cleaner and smaller pores, exfoliation, higher energy levels, and it can even help reduce cellulite.

Spend More Time in Nature

Spending time in nature helps you feel relaxed while getting much-needed fresh air. Because of this, you should spend as much time as possible in nature and in the great outdoors. If you allow yourself to relax as part of your juice cleanse, you may want to spend most of your time outdoors. If you have nothing to do at home or at work, go to your local park for some fresh air. You can even spend time in your own garden to meditate, sit in silence or even do some light gardening.

Switch Your Products

As you start choosing organic fruits and veggies for your juicing journey, you can go beyond this by switching the other products in your home too. Check your cleaning supplies, laundry detergents, and even your cosmetics to see if these contain any unwanted or harmful chemicals. Change these products to organic ones that don't contain any chemicals. This will help reduce your risk of getting chemicals in your system to make it easier for your body to detoxify itself naturally.

Take the Right Supplements

Although following a healthy and balanced diet while juicing can already improve your health immensely, you may choose to take supplements too. Such supplements can be very beneficial, especially if you want to avoid nutrient deficiencies. But before you take supplements, have a conversation with your doctor first. Have your nutrient levels checked and ask your doctor about the best supplements you should take for your overall health. Some examples of supplements that you can take along with your healthy diet are probiotics, spirulina, omega-3, omega-6, and omega-9.

Reduce Your Caloric Intake

If you want to lose weight, then this tip is for you. Since you will be supplementing your diet with juicing, then you may start reducing your caloric intake. Drinking a glass of fresh juice half an hour before your meals can make this easier for you as you will feel fuller afterward. Another way to do this is by replacing your snacks with smoothies or juice blends—but only replace your snacks, not your meals. Do this gradually so you don't feel like you are restricting yourself. Also, remember to listen to your body to avoid getting sick or experiencing any adverse health issues.

Improve the Way You Eat

In line with the previous point, you can also learn how to improve the way you eat. There are several ways to do this such as:

- Keeping your portion sizes small and eating regularly throughout the day. This prevents you from overeating.
- Chew your food thoroughly so that your body can digest it easily.
- Vary the foods you eat so that you don't end up craving for certain foods. If you have a varied diet, you will feel

more interested in sticking with your healthy, balanced diet.

- Try to eat whole fruits and veggies, even the ones you are not particularly fond of. The more you eat them, the more you will get used to them.
- Learn how to eat mindfully. Having awareness while eating gives you a chance to learn how to listen to your body better.

Your diet should never be something you feel stressed about. It should be something that nourishes you, keeps you alive, and makes you feel happy. And when you add juicing to your diet, this will make it even better

-

Conclusion: Ready, Set, Juice!

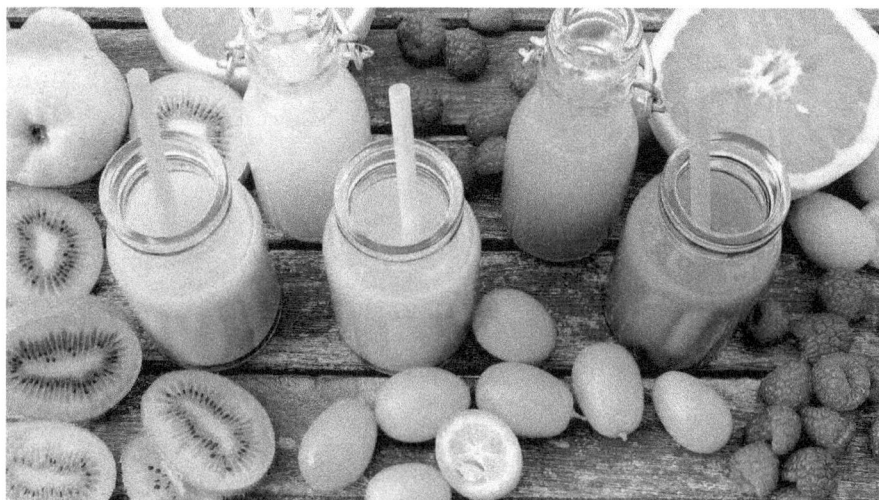

Fig. 20: Time to Juice. Pixabay, by silviarita, 2017,
https://pixabay.com/photos/smoothies-fruits-colorful-vitamins-2253423/ Copyright 2017 by
silviarita/Pixabay.

There you have it!

Everything you need to know about juicing. By now, you are
already armed with the information you need to start your own
juicing journey safely and correctly. As promised at the beginning
of the book, I shared with you everything I learned and
discovered throughout my juicing journey. We started this eBook
by defining what juicing is, answered the most important
question related to juicing, discussed the benefits of juicing, and
you even learned the most important things to keep in mind
when you start juicing. The next chapter was all about finding the
perfect juicer. Here, you learned all about the different types of
juicers along with the whole process of how to find the best
juicer for your needs.

In the next chapter, you learned all about preparing the ingredients you need for your juices. Here, you learned the best fruits and vegetables to juice along with the most challenging ones. This chapter also contained very helpful and practical information about how to prepare ingredients, and what you can do with the pulp, seeds, and peels of your fruits and veggies after juicing. If you want to make juicing a permanent part of your life, you can even start growing your own produce. If this is something that you might be interested in, you should consider getting the next book about greenhouse gardening in the series. This book is all about year-round plant growing in a greenhouse, advanced techniques, wintertime maintenance specifics, and more. With your own garden, it would be much more economical for you to make juicing a regular part of your life.

Going back to our eBook, the next two chapters were all about weight loss. The first chapter was about how juicing promotes weight loss and how you can enjoy this benefit by juicing properly. The next chapter contained a bunch of tasty, healthy, and simple recipes that you can start making right now. More recipes followed in the next chapter but this time, these recipes helped promote other health benefits of juicing. In the seventh chapter, you learned all about juice cleanses. It even contained a simple plan for you to follow a 3-day juice cleanse (if you're a beginner) and a 7-day juice cleanse (if you're more experienced). And in the last chapter, you learned all about the lifestyle changes you can make to enhance your juicing journey.

In this eBook, you discovered a wealth of information about juicing—more than enough to make you a juicing expert. Now, all you have to do is apply what you have learned by embarking on your own juicing journey. When you do your first juice cleanse, you will already know how to do it safely and correctly. If you enjoyed reading this eBook as much as I enjoyed writing it, please leave a review on Amazon. That way, other people who are interested in juicing can also learn what they need to improve their health. Now that you have reached the end, it's time for you to take action. Good luck and happy juicing!

References

Absolutely Flavorful. (2020, February 21). *WHAT TO JUICE FOR GUT HEALTH*. Absolutely Flavorful. https://absolutelyflavorful.com/what-to-juice-for-gut-he alth-2/

Andrews, R. (2014, January 22). *Detox diets. Juice cleanses. Could they be making you more toxic?* Precision Nutrition. https://www.precisionnutrition.com/detox-cleanse-diets

Arora, S. (2018, March 28). *The 7-Day Detox Diet Plan: Time to Get Healthy & Active*. NDTV Food. https://food.ndtv.com/health/tthe-7-day-detox-diet-time -to-get-healthy-active-1267044

Atkins, R. (2017, January 15). *Detox Juicing for Weight Loss - Quick & Easy Diet Tips*. Vitality 4 Life. https://www.vitality4life.co.uk/blog/healthy-lifestyle/los e-weight-juicing

Bennett, B. (2016, May 24). *Omega J8006 Nutrition Center Juicer review*. CNET. https://www.cnet.com/reviews/omega-j8006-nutrition-c enter-juicer-review/

Bennett, B. (2020a, April 29). *8 Dos and Don'ts for Using Your Juicer*. CNET. https://www.cnet.com/how-to/how-to-juice-at-home-jui cer-tips/

Bennett, B. (2020b, April 29). *How to Pick the Right Juicer*. CNET. https://www.cnet.com/how-to/how-to-pick-the-right-jui cer/

Best Juicer Reviews Guide. (2020, January 1). *Breville Juice Fountain Juicer – JE98XL The Ultimate Best Fast Juicer Of 2020*. Best

Juicer   Reviews.
http://bestjuicerreviewsguides.com/breville-juice-fountai
n-juicer/

Bhatnagar, S. (2018, April 6). *Vegetable Juices: 6 Interesting Health And Beauty Benefits.* NDTV Food. https://food.ndtv.com/food-drinks/vegetable-juices-6-in teresting-health-and-beauty-benefits-1833709

Biswas, D. (2013, October 10). *Best Fruit Juice Recipes to Fight Aging - Natural Foods for Skin.* The Fit Indian. https://www.thefitindian.com/blog/best-fruit-juice-recip es-to-fight-anti-aging/

Boldt, A. (n.d.). *Will Juicing Help Me to Lose Weight?* LIVESTRONG. https://www.livestrong.com/article/224906-will-juicing- help-me-to-lose-weight/

Boldt, A. (2019a, May 31). *How to Drink Grapefruit Juice to Lose Weight.* LIVESTRONG. https://www.livestrong.com/article/213562-how-to-drin k-grapefruit-juice-to-lose-weight/

Boldt, A. (2019b, May 31). *How to Drink Grapefruit Juice to Lose Weight.* LIVESTRONG. https://www.livestrong.com/article/213562-how-to-drin k-grapefruit-juice-to-lose-weight/

Bowker, S. (2019, April 30). *Carrot Juice Recipe for Weight Loss.* Cultured   Palate. https://myculturedpalate.com/carrot-juice-recipe-for-wei ght-loss/

Bren. (2018, January 11). *How To Do A 10 Day Juice Fast: A Monster Guide.* Bren on The Road. https://brenontheroad.com/10-day-juice-fast/

Brigette, F. (2014, August 15). *6 Tips For Juicing At Home.* Free People   Blog.

https://blog.freepeople.com/2014/08/6-tips-juicing-ho
me/

Brown, M. J. (2019, October 4). *Juicing: Good or Bad?* Healthline.
https://www.healthline.com/nutrition/juicing-good-or-b
ad

Brown, N. (2015, May 26). *How to Juice Your Way to a Healthy
Lifestyle.* Fix.
https://www.fix.com/blog/juice-your-way-to-a-healthier-
lifestyle/

Bryant, A. (n.d.). *Anita Bryant Quote.* Quotefancy.
https://quotefancy.com/quote/1631521/Anita-Bryant-B
reakfast-without-orange-juice-is-like-a-day-without-sunshi
ne

Butler, N. (2018, September 20). *Juicing vs. Blending: Which Is Better
for Me?* Healthline.
https://www.healthline.com/health/food-nutrition/juici
ng-vs-blending

Carey, S. (2015, April 19). *What Kinds Of Exercises Can You Do
During A Juice Cleanse?* Raw Juice Cleanse Recipes.
https://www.rawjuicecleanserecipes.com/blog/2015/04/
19/what-kinds-of-exercises-can-you-do-during-a-juice-cle
anse/

Carter, R. (n.d.). *15 Juicing Recipes for Weight Loss.* Best Blender
USA.
https://www.bestblenderusa.com/juicing-recipes-for-wei
ght-loss/

Cole, W. (2016, October 10). *3 Flavorful Drink Recipes To Help
Balance Thyroid, Adrenal & Reproductive Hormone Function.*
Mindbodygreen.
https://www.mindbodygreen.com/0-26873/3-elixirs-to-b
oost-your-thyroid-adrenal-sex-hormones.html

Coles, L. T., & Clifton, P. M. (2012). Effect of beetroot juice on
lowering blood pressure in free-living, disease-free adults:

a randomized, placebo-controlled trial. *Nutrition Journal*, *11*(1). https://doi.org/10.1186/1475-2891-11-106

Colquhoun, J. (n.d.). *Are You Making These 8 Common Juicing Mistakes?* Hungry For Change. http://www.hungryforchange.tv/article/are-you-making-these-common-8-juicing-mistakes

Consumer Select. (2018). *How to Choose a Juicer For Your Juicing Needs.* Consumer Select Juicers. http://www.consumerselect.org/how-to-choose-a-juicer/

Cooks, M. (2015, October 11). *Preparing Vegetables for Juicing + Root Vegetable Juice Recipe.* Ben and Me. https://www.benandme.com/preparing-vegetables-for-juicing/

Cross, J. (2019). *Produce Prep.* Joe Cross. https://www.rebootwithjoe.com/juicing/produce-prep/

Dai, Q., Borenstein, A. R., Wu, Y., Jackson, J. C., & Larson, E. B. (2006). Fruit and Vegetable Juices and Alzheimer's Disease: The Kame Project. *The American Journal of Medicine*, *119*(9), 751–759. https://doi.org/10.1016/j.amjmed.2006.03.045

Dalkin, G. (2016, January 5). *Juice Cleanse 101.* What's Gaby Cooking. https://whatsgabycooking.com/juice-cleanse-2/

Daws, M. (2016, September 26). *10 Shocking Health Benefits of Juicing, With Recipes!* Lifehack. https://www.lifehack.org/374413/10-shocking-health-benefits-of-juicing-with-recipes

de Bellefonds, C. (2019, October 29). *What You Should Know Before Trying Juicing for Weight Loss.* Men's Health. https://www.menshealth.com/nutrition/a29623273/juicing-for-weight-loss/

Dershin, A. (2017). *How to Exercise on a Juice Cleanse.* THE GOOD CLUB.

https://www.getgood.club/archives/2019/8/6/how-to-e
xercise-on-a-juice-cleanse

Doctor Oz. (2020). *The Healing Properties of Juicing.* Doctor Oz.
https://www.doctoroz.com/article/healing-properties-jui
cing

Doman, E. (2015, October 9). *8 Reasons You Should Start Juicing.*
Compact   Appliance.
https://learn.compactappliance.com/juicing-benefits/

Doustdar, R. (2017). *Veggies vs. Fruits.* Everyday Juicer.
http://www.everydayjuicer.com/veggies-vs-fruits

Elliott, B. (2016, November 30). *Can Juicing Help You Lose Weight?*
Healthline.
https://www.healthline.com/nutrition/can-juicing-help-y
ou-lose-weight

Esfahani, A., Wong, J. M. W., Truan, J., Villa, C. R., Mirrahimi,
A., Srichaikul, K., & Kendall, C. W. C. (2011). Health
Effects of Mixed Fruit and Vegetable Concentrates: A
Systematic Review of the Clinical Interventions. *Journal of
the American College of Nutrition*, *30*(5), 285–294.
https://doi.org/10.1080/07315724.2011.10719971

Eske, J. (2019, February 28). *Top 3 juices to relieve constipation, why
they work, and recipes.* Medical News Today.
https://www.medicalnewstoday.com/articles/324585

Fey, R. (2020, June 7). *How to Do a Juice Cleanse.* Goodnature.
https://www.goodnature.com/blog/how-to-do-a-juice-cl
eanse/#recipes

Food Babe. (2013, August 6). *Are You Making These Common Juicing
Mistakes?* Food Babe.
https://foodbabe.com/juicing-mistakes/

Fulgoni, V. L., Keast, D. R., Bailey, R. L., & Dwyer, J. (2011).
Foods, Fortificants, and Supplements: Where Do
Americans Get Their Nutrients? *The Journal of Nutrition*,

141(10), 1847–1854. https://doi.org/10.3945/jn.111.142257

Gajendran, D. (2015, February 11). *10 Amazing Natural Juices for Improving Digestive Health*. The Fit Indian. https://www.thefitindian.com/blog/healthy-digestive-juices/#Green-Apple-Kale-and-Cucumber-Smoothie

Georgiou, C. (2015, October 19). *How Juicing Helps Balance Hormones*. Joe Cross. https://www.rebootwithjoe.com/how-juicing-helps-balance-hormones/

Gibson, A., Edgar, J. D., Neville, C. E., Gilchrist, S. E., McKinley, M. C., Patterson, C. C., Young, I. S., & Woodside, J. V. (2012). Effect of fruit and vegetable consumption on immune function in older people: a randomized controlled trial. *The American Journal of Clinical Nutrition, 96*(6), 1429–1436. https://doi.org/10.3945/ajcn.112.039057

Goodnature. (2020a, February 15). *3-Day DIY Juice Cleanse (Recipes, Benefits & Tips)*. Goodnature. https://www.goodnature.com/blog/3-day-diy-juice-cleanse/

Goodnature. (2020b, March 8). *How to Juice Fast Safely: 9 Tips for Success*. Goodnature. https://www.goodnature.com/blog/how-to-juice-fast-safely-9-tips-for-success/

Goodnature. (2020c, March 8). *How to Juice Fast Safely: 9 Tips for Success*. Goodnature. https://www.goodnature.com/blog/how-to-juice-fast-safely-9-tips-for-success/

Hannum, C. (2019, July 5). *Burn Fat With Watermelon Juice*. The Spruce Eats. https://www.thespruceeats.com/watermelon-juice-recipe-to-burn-fat-2078407

Harrington, M. (2018, February 12). *A Guide to Smoothie and Juice Supplements*. Azumio. https://www.azumio.com/blog/nutrition/a-guide-to-smoothie-juice-supplements

Healthy Juicers. (2017). *A Comprehensive Guide On How To Choose A Juicer*. Healthy Wise Choice. https://healthywisechoice.com/a-comprehensive-guide-on-how-to-choose-a-juicer/

HEB. (2020). Heb.Com. https://www.heb.com/recipe/recipe-article/how-to-juice-fruits-vegetables/1398804484658

Hendricks, J. (n.d.). *Cucumber Juice for Weight Loss*. LIVESTRONG. https://www.livestrong.com/article/303776-cucumber-juice-for-weight-loss/

Henning, S. M., Yang, J., Shao, P., Lee, R.-P., Huang, J., Ly, A., Hsu, M., Lu, Q.-Y., Thames, G., Heber, D., & Li, Z. (2017). Health benefit of vegetable/fruit juice-based diet: Role of microbiome. *Scientific Reports*, *7*(1). https://doi.org/10.1038/s41598-017-02200-6

Hicks, K. (2015, August 7). *How to Buy the Best Juicer For You*. Compact Appliance. https://learn.compactappliance.com/juicer-buyers-guide/

Holland, K. (2019, July 2). *How to Choose the Right Types of Juicers for You*. Real Simple. https://www.realsimple.com/food-recipes/tools-products/appliances/types-of-juicers

Holmes, E. (2015, April 21). *13 Detox Juices To Drink Yourself Clean*. Mindbodygreen. https://www.mindbodygreen.com/0-18335/13-detox-juices-to-drink-yourself-clean.html

Holthaus, T. (2020). *The Do's and Don'ts of Juicing.* Foxy. https://foxy.com/blog/the-dos-and-donts-of-juicing

How To Do a Juice Cleanse. (2015). Project Juice. https://www.projectjuice.com/how-to-cleanse

Hulburt, J. (2016, May 4). *3 Juice and Smoothie Recipes to Balance Hormones.* WILD Wellness. http://www.jennihulburt.com/2016/05/3-juice-and-smoothie-recipes-to-balance-hormones/

Jessica. (2014, January 29). *Top 10 Health Benefits Of Juicing.* Live The Life You Love. https://www.ilivethelifeilove.com/health-benefits-of-juicing/

John Wiley & Sons. (2020). *How to Choose the Best Juicer for You: A Buying Guide.* Dummies. https://www.dummies.com/home-garden/juicer-buying-guide/

Johns, A. (2017, February 2). *10 Detox Juice Recipes for Weight Loss Cleanse | Juice Cleanse.* Lose Weight By Eating. https://loseweightbyeating.com/10-detox-juice-recipes-weight-loss-cleanse/

Juicer Kitchen. (2015, September 3). *31 Reasons Why You Should Start Juicing Right Now.* Juicer Kitchen. https://juicer.kitchen/31-reasons-to-start-juicing/

Just on Juice. (2015a). *3 Day Juice Fast Plan.* JustonJuice. http://www.justonjuice.com/3-day-juice-fast-plan/

Just on Juice. (2015b). *7 Day Juice Fast Plan.* JustonJuice. http://www.justonjuice.com/7-day-juice-fast-plan/

Kastashchuk, A. (2014, October 7). *Benefits of Juice Fasting.* Fresh Start. https://www.healthretreat.ca/healthy-lifestyle/benefits-of-juice-fasting/

Kathrin. (2019a, May 9). *Juicing for Hormonal Imbalance – Two Powerful Yet Simple Recipes.* MyHIRSUTISM. https://myhirsutism.com/juicing-for-hormonal-imbalance/

Kent RO Systems. (2017, March 8). *Cold Pressed Juicer (Slow Juicer) Buying Guide 2019.* Kent Healthcare Products. https://www.kent.co.in/blog/cold-pressed-juicer-buying-guide/

Knudsen, M. (2013, January 9). *Juice Fasting: The Right (And Wrong) Way To Do Your Cleanse, According To A Nutritionist.* Mindbodygreen. https://www.mindbodygreen.com/0-7334/the-right-and-wrong-way-to-juice.html

Kogler, C. (2016, April 8). *Here's What You Should Eat Right After a Juice Cleanse.* The Daily Meal. https://www.thedailymeal.com/healthy-eating/here-s-what-you-should-eat-right-after-juice-cleanse-slideshow/slide-9

Lidder, S., & Webb, A. J. (2013). Vascular effects of dietary nitrate (as found in green leafy vegetables and beetroot) via the nitrate-nitrite-nitric oxide pathway. *British Journal of Clinical Pharmacology, 75*(3), 677–696. https://doi.org/10.1111/j.1365-2125.2012.04420.x

Link, R. (2019, July 4). *The 12 Best Vegetables to Juice.* Healthline. https://www.healthline.com/nutrition/best-vegetables-to-juice

Lokshin, E., & Yuen, C. (2020, June 5). *10 Tasty Beverages to Boost Your Immune System.* Healthline. https://www.healthline.com/health/juice-immune-system-boost

Magdalen, L. (2019, December 27). *Best Fruits and Vegetables to Juice.* CompuKitchen. https://compukitchen.com/best-fruits-and-vegetables-to-juice/

Maleh, J. (n.d.-a). *7 Tips That Will Make Your Juice Cleanse Easier.* Jus By Julie. https://www.jusbyjulie.com/blogs/news/7-tips-that-will-make-your-juice-cleanse-easier

Maleh, J. (n.d.-b). *Sip + Sweat: The Best Workouts for When You're On a Juice Cleanse.* Jus By Julie. https://www.jusbyjulie.com/blogs/news/sip-sweat-the-b est-workouts-for-when-youre-on-a-juice-cleanse

Masterson, F., & Girdwain, J. (2019a, September 13). *Juice Recipes You'll Love–No Matter How You Feel About Juicing for Health.* Shape. https://www.shape.com/healthy-eating/healthy-drinks/b est-juice-whats-bugging-you

Masterson, F., & Girdwain, J. (2019b, September 13). *Juice Recipes You'll Love–No Matter How You Feel About Juicing for Health.* Shape. https://www.shape.com/healthy-eating/healthy-drinks/b est-juice-whats-bugging-you?slide=893d2902-8d02-4961-946b-f46c49eda2e8#893d2902-8d02-4961-946b-f46c49ed a2e8

MaxLiving. (n.d.). *How to Go on a Healthy Juice Cleanse.* MaxLiving. https://maxliving.com/healthy-articles/how-to-juice-clea nse/

May, D. (2016, January 20). *7 Ways to Use Your Leftover Juice Pulp.* HuffPost. https://www.huffpost.com/entry/7-ways-to-use-your-lef tover-juice-pulp_b_9028296

Meghawache, B. (2017). *Juicing 101.* Nourished by Bri. https://www.nourishedbybri.com/juicing-101

Mills, M. (2016, November 18). *7 Refreshing Drinks that Lower Your Blood Pressure.* Vive Health. https://www.vivehealth.com/blogs/resources/drinks-tha t-lower-blood-pressure

Mohla, D. (2018, February 1). *6 Power Fruits You Should Include in Your Diet to Detox.* NDTV Food. https://food.ndtv.com/food-drinks/6-power-fruits-you-should-include-in-your-diet-to-detox-1677523

Mukherjee, S. (2019, November 19). *10 Amazing Benefits Of Drinking Vegetable Juices For Health And Beauty.* STYLECRAZE. https://www.stylecraze.com/articles/amazing-benefits-of-drinking-vegetable-juices-for-health-and-beauty/

Nall, R. (2018, September 21). *What are the Pros and Cons of a Juice Cleanse?* Medical News Today. https://www.medicalnewstoday.com/articles/323136

NDTV Food. (2019, February 13). *10 Fat Burning Juices You Must Have for Quick Weight Loss.* NDTV Food. https://food.ndtv.com/health/10-juices-you-must-have-for-quick-weight-loss-1669424

NDTV Food Desk. (2018, October 15). *Weight Loss: Here's How Drinking Pomegranate (Anaar) Juice Daily May Help Weight Loss.* NDTV. https://www.ndtv.com/food/weight-loss-heres-how-drinking-pomegranate-anaar-juice-daily-may-help-weight-loss-1931523

NDTV Food Desk. (2019a, October 3). *Weight Loss: Drinking Cabbage Juice May Help Lose Weight And Burn Body Fat.* NDTV. https://www.ndtv.com/food/weight-loss-drinking-cabbage-juice-may-help-lose-weight-and-burn-body-fat-1952769

NDTV Food Desk. (2019b, October 21). *Hypertension: 3 Vegetable Juices To Manage High Blood Pressure.* NDTV. https://www.ndtv.com/food/hypertension-3-vegetable-juices-to-manage-high-blood-pressure-1906095

Nguyen, A. (2014, February 25). *Juicing for Health and Weight Loss.* WebMD.

https://www.webmd.com/diet/features/juicing-health-ri
sks-and-benefits#1

Orecchio, C. (2018, April 12). *Juice Reset: 7 Day Raw Food & Juice Cleanse.* The Whole Journey. https://thewholejourney.com/7-day-juice-cleanse/

Papantoniou, N. (2020, June 12). *This Adorable Citrus Juicer Is the Perfect Addition to Your Bar Cart.* Good Housekeeping. https://www.goodhousekeeping.com/appliances/juicer-r eviews/g598/best-juicers/

Pasquale, N. (2013, March 12). *How to Do a Juice Cleanse.* Urban Remedy. https://urbanremedy.com/how-to-do-a-juice-cleanse/

Pressed Juicery. (2019, October 24). *How To Do a Juice Cleanse.* Pressed Juicery. https://pressedjuicery.com/blogs/pressed-life/juice-clea nse-guide

Price, M. (2020, July 3). *The Best Juicers for 2020.* CNET. https://www.cnet.com/news/best-vpn-service-in-2020-e xpressvpn-nordvpn-surfshark-and-more/

Purmalek, M. (2013, August 8). *6 Things You Need to Know About Juicing Your Veggies.* National Center for Health Research. http://www.center4research.org/6-things-need-know-jui cing-veggies/

Regina, L. (2020, January 24). *Best Juicers of 2020 – The Ultimate Buying Guide & Reviews.* Healthy Kitchen 101. https://healthykitchen101.com/best-juicers/

Robbins, J. (2017, November 1). *5 Tips For Juicing Correctly | Robbins Natural Health Specialists.* Robbins Natural Health. https://drjoelrobbins.com/5-juicing-tips/

Sanders, H. (2018, February 1). *The 3 Best Juicing Recipes for Blood Pressure.* Health Ambition. https://www.healthambition.com/juicing-recipes-blood-pressure/

Sara. (2019b, January 9). *3 Healthy Immunity Boosting Juices.* The Bettered Blondie. https://thebetteredblondie.com/3-healthy-immunity-boosting-juices/

Satrazemis, E. (2019, May 15). *Juicing for Weight Loss: The Pros and Cons.* Trifecta. https://www.trifectanutrition.com/blog/juicing-for-weight-loss-the-pros-and-cons

Schiller, N. (2018, April 12). *19 Superfood Add-Ins for Power-Packed Smoothies & Juices.* Foodal. https://foodal.com/drinks-2/smoothies/superfood-add-ins/

Shain, S. (2013, February 20). *How to Do a 3-Day DIY Juice Cleanse: Recipes & Strategy.* Susan Shain. https://susanshain.com/3-day-diy-juice-cleanse-for-travelers/

Sharp, A. (2018, August 15). *The Foods That Balance Out (or Mess With) Your Hormones.* Greatist. https://greatist.com/eat/foods-for-hormonal-imbalance#1

Spritzler, F. (2019, April 17). *14 Simple Ways to Stick to a Healthy Diet.* Healthline. https://www.healthline.com/nutrition/14-ways-to-stick-to-a-diet

Stadler, M. (2018, September 18). *Healthy Juice Cleanse Recipes.* Modern Honey. https://www.modernhoney.com/healthy-juice-cleanse-recipes/

Susan, R. (2015, November 2). *Juicing For Weight Loss and Health.* What's Cooking America. https://whatscookingamerica.net/Information/JuicingWeightLoss.htm

The Steaming Pot. (2017, May 4). *Juicing Recipes: 7-Day Plan.* The Steaming Pot. https://www.steamingpot.com/juicing-recipes-7-day-plan/

TheLifeCo. (n.d.). *After Detox Diet.* The LifeCo: Detox and Wellness Centers. Retrieved August 6, 2020, from https://www.thelifeco.com/en/after-detox-diet/

Vartan, S. (2019, January 2). *How to Choose a Juicer.* Treehugger. https://www.treehugger.com/how-to-choose-a-juicer-or-do-you-need-a-blender-4860205

Vemb, C. (2019, November 15). *What To Eat After A Juice Cleanse.* Pulp & Press Juice Co. https://www.pulpandpress.com/what-to-eat-after-juice-cleanse/

Waldman, S. (2017, April 1). *The Beginner's Guide to Making Juice.* The Week. https://theweek.com/articles/688700/beginners-guide-making-juice

Well Pared. (2017, October 26). *13 Ways A Juice Cleanse Can Boost Your Health.* Well Pared. https://wellpared.com/13-ways-juice-cleanse-can-boost-health/

What Vegetables & Fruits Should Not Be Juiced? (2020). Extreme Wellness Supply. https://extremewellnesssupply.com/blogs/news/what-vegetables-fruits-should-not-be-juiced

Wong, C. (2020a, February 3). *How to End a Cleanse Safely.* Verywell Fit. https://www.verywellfit.com/how-to-end-a-cleanse-89112

Wong, C. (2020b, February 4). *What Is a Juice Cleanse?* Verywell Fit. https://www.verywellfit.com/juice-cleanse-89120

Zeratsky, K. (2016). *What to Know Before You Juice*. Mayo Clinic. https://www.mayoclinic.org/healthy-lifestyle/nutrition-and-healthy-eating/expert-answers/juicing/faq-20058020

Zeratsky, K. (2019, October 1). *Is Juicing Healthier Than Eating Whole Fruits or Vegetables?* Mayo Clinic. https://www.mayoclinic.org/healthy-lifestyle/nutrition-and-healthy-eating/expert-answers/juicing/faq-20058020#:~:text=They%20say%20juicing%20can%20reduce

www.ingramcontent.com/pod-product-compliance
Lightning Source LLC
Chambersburg PA
CBHW031120020426

42333CB00012B/169